EYE AND VISION RESEARCH DEVELOPMENTS

EYE MOVEMENT DISORDERS (NYSTAGMUS AND STRABISMUS)

DIAGNOSIS, MANAGEMENT AND IMPACT ON QUALITY OF LIFE

EYE AND VISION RESEARCH DEVELOPMENTS

Additional books in this series can be found on Nova's website under the Series tab.

Additional e-books in this series can be found on Nova's website under the e-book tab.

EYE AND VISION RESEARCH DEVELOPMENTS

EYE MOVEMENT DISORDERS (NYSTAGMUS AND STRABISMUS)

DIAGNOSIS, MANAGEMENT AND IMPACT ON QUALITY OF LIFE

SLOAN L. MILLS
EDITOR

New York

For permission to use material from this book please contact us:
Telephone 631-231-7269; Fax 631-231-8175
Web Site: http://www.novapublishers.com

Library of Congress Cataloging-in-Publication Data

ISBN: 978-1-63321-980-9

Library of Congress Control Number: 2014949886

Published by Nova Science Publishers, Inc. † New York

Contents

Preface

The anesthetic implications of eye muscle surgery are varied and numerous. Being a condition that can be seen in all age groups, the anesthetist or anesthesiologist will see pediatric, adult, and geriatric patient populations. This book examines and analyzes the causes, symptoms and treatment options to strabismus and nystagmus. It discusses benign paroxysmal positional vertigo; strabismus surgery; central positional dizziness; the treatment of intermittent exotropia in childhood; and nystagmus in posterior fossa stroke patients.

Chapter 1 – Benign paroxysmal positional vertigo (BPPV) is one of the most common disorders of the vestibular system. Its one-year incidence is 0.6%, and its lifetime prevalence is 2.4%. Although the majority of individuals with BPPV are females over the age of 50, an individual's health-related quality of life is negatively affected regardless of gender or age. BPPV is often associated with anxiety and depression; and it may lead to falls, especially in older adults, because of its impact upon both static and dynamic postural control. The primary cause of BPPV is believed to be the aging process. However, traumatic brain injuries and inner ear diseases may also induce the signs and symptoms of BPPV, especially in individuals under the age of 50. BPPV occurs when otoconia become detached from the utricle of the affected inner ear and travel into one of the semicircular canals. If the otoconia remain free floating in the endolymph of that particular semicircular canal, this condition is known as canalolithiasis. If the otoconia become attached to the cupula of that particular semicircular canal, this condition is known as cupulolithiasis. Because otoconia have been known to travel into all three semicircular canals, the specific types of BPPV are posterior (or inferior) canal BPPV, anterior (or superior) canal BPPV, and lateral (or horizontal) canal

BPPV. This chapter will discuss (a) an overview of the vestibular system; (b) an overview of BPPV, including the characteristics of the nystagmus associated with each type of BPPV; (c) the methods used to evaluate each type of BPPV; and (d) the methods used to treat each type of BPPV.

Chapter 2 – The anesthetic implications of eye muscle surgery are varied and numerous. Being a condition that can be seen in all age groups, the anesthetist or anesthesiologist will see pediatric, adult, and geriatric patient populations. Though it may be minimally invasive on an anatomical basis, strabismus surgery can be perhaps surprisingly invasive physiologically because of the oculocardiac reflex, and the clinician needs to be well versed in management and treatment of any cardiac dysrhythmia so that if it occurs, it can be handled instantly and successfully. Since eye muscle surgery is usually done on an outpatient basis, post-operative nausea and vomiting need to be well controlled even though eye muscle surgery is well known for being very nausea-provoking. Our chapter will focus on these factors in detail.

Chapter 3 – While positional dizziness is most commonly related to peripheral vestibular disease, it may rarely be caused by a pontomedullary or vestibulocerebellar lesion. Three main clinical forms have been described: central positional nystagmus (CPN), central paroxysmal positional vertigo (CPPV), and rotational vertebral artery syndrome (RVAS). The first type consists of prolonged positional nystagmus with no or only slight vertigo (e.g. pure downbeat nystagmus in head-hanging position) and seems to be precipitated by a strategic lesion in the cerebellar nodulus and uvula. The second type comprises short-lasting nystagmus combined with vertigo and is provoked by lesions dorsolateral to the fourth ventricle, in the cerebellar vermis or superior cerebellar peduncle. The mechanism by which such lesions cause positional nystagmus seems to involve a vestibular tone imbalance promoted by disruption of the central otolithic connections between the vestibular nuclei and vestibular cerebellum. Typical causes for CPN and CPPV include haemorrhage, tumour, demyelination, infarction, Chiari malformation and cerebellar degeneration. Vestibular migraine and drug intoxication should also be considered, especially when imaging is normal. The main differential diagnosis of CPPV is benign paroxysmal positional vertigo (BPPV), and given the potentially serious prognosis of infratentorial lesions, this is a critical distinction. Positional nystagmus beating in a plane inconsistent with head and semicircular canal stimulation or purely vertical or torsional should raise suspicion of a central lesion; other features that favor a central origin include absent latency, fatigability and habituation on repetitive stimulation, positional or positioning nystagmus without vertigo, positioning-induced vomiting without nystagmus, and additional cerebellar and oculomotor signs. A third type of central positional dizziness is caused by dynamic compression of one vertebral artery as a result of head rotation (RVAS) promoting transient ischemia of the cerebellum and/or labyrinth, with resultant nystagmus and vertigo. Untreated RVAS may lead to posterior circulation stroke.

Chapter 4 – This study presents 124 children aged less than 15 years suffering from a temporary divergent squint when looking into the far distance. These children were treated and observed in an ophthalmologist's office over the past 35 years. No evidence-based rules for treating intermittent divergent squints are found in the literature. The possibilities are: (1) Prescription of glasses, (2) Short-term occlusion of one eye against suppression, (3) Orthoptic exercises, (4) Prismatic correction of the squint over some years, (5) Surgery, and (6) Contact lenses in older and myopic children.

The aim of treatment is to establish a steady compensated exophoria with a latent angle as small as possible; in rare cases the result may be orthophoria. The patients sample showed some specific characteristics: 44.5% started squinting in the 2nd and 3rd year of life, 76.6% had unilateral strabismus and suppression, but no severe amblyopia and - 67% had approximate emmetropia, which played a role in compliance with wearing glasses. Most ophthalmologists prefer to wait and observe the child for some time; if the child's squint deteriorates, an operation will be proposed. The success of such operations is uncertain. I adopted a conservative treatment approach starting with prisms. Unlike older children the younger children – aged less than 10 years – mostly accepted the glasses necessary to apply the press-on-prisms which correct the squint angle for distance. After a short time, the eye position fixing near objects relaxes and the children had almost the same squint deviation for near and distant fixation. Therefore the diagnosis was "pseudodivergence excess" in almost all the children, only two had convergence insufficiency and two others needed bifocals. In periodical controls, the prisms were adapted to the current eye position. In this way, - in spite of squint – fusion was trained throughout the day and suppression eliminated. Step-by-step the squint angle decreased, with a reduction of on average 13Δ, and finally, after average 4.3 years the prisms could be removed. The longer the time of prism-treatment, the more constant was the result, even after years. This method is recommended only for children with a squint deviation of up to 10°. More severe squints require surgery; but the results are better after preparation of the binocular functions by prisms. A small postoperative divergence can be treated again with prisms or with contact lenses in cases of myopia.

The therapy should be started as soon as possible after the onset of the squint, as the recovery time will be less. Parents should be warned that treatment takes a long time. However, treatment is safe and results in good sensorial preconditions for adult life.

Chapter 5 – In this chapter the authors will describe briefly the pathophysiological mechanisms of central nystagmus generation, proceed with the description of bedside examination of the patient with sudden onset of vertigo and unsteadiness. They will present the results of 9 patients with stroke diagnosis who were during the year 2013 admitted to our Neurological Emergency Department and who came with sudden onset of vertigo and unsteadiness as the leading symptom of illness. On the basis of these results the authors will discuss the importance of recognition of the impairment of central vestibular pathways as solely symptoms or additional symptoms in the early diagnosis of cerebral stroke. The therapeutic guidelines will be presented as well.

In: Eye Movement Disorders
Editor: Sloan L. Mills

ISBN: 978-1-63321-980-9

Chapter 1

Benign Paroxysmal Positional Vertigo

Bonni L. Kinne, PT, MSPT, MA[*]
Grand Valley State University, Allendale, Michigan, US

Abstract

Benign paroxysmal positional vertigo (BPPV) is one of the most common disorders of the vestibular system. Its one-year incidence is 0.6%, and its lifetime prevalence is 2.4%. Although the majority of individuals with BPPV are females over the age of 50, an individual's health-related quality of life is negatively affected regardless of gender or age. BPPV is often associated with anxiety and depression; and it may lead to falls, especially in older adults, because of its impact upon both static and dynamic postural control. The primary cause of BPPV is believed to be the aging process. However, traumatic brain injuries and inner ear diseases may also induce the signs and symptoms of BPPV, especially in individuals under the age of 50. BPPV occurs when otoconia become detached from the utricle of the affected inner ear and travel into one of the semicircular canals. If the otoconia remain free floating in the endolymph of that particular semicircular canal, this condition is known as canalolithiasis. If the otoconia become attached to the cupula of that particular semicircular canal, this condition is known as

[*] Corresponding author: Email: kinneb@gvsu.edu.

cupulolithiasis. Because otoconia have been known to travel into all three semicircular canals, the specific types of BPPV are posterior (or inferior) canal BPPV, anterior (or superior) canal BPPV, and lateral (or horizontal) canal BPPV. This chapter will discuss (a) an overview of the vestibular system; (b) an overview of BPPV, including the characteristics of the nystagmus associated with each type of BPPV; (c) the methods used to evaluate each type of BPPV; and (d) the methods used to treat each type of BPPV.

Introduction

Benign paroxysmal positional vertigo (BPPV) is one of the most common disorders of the vestibular system. Its one-year incidence is 0.6%, and its lifetime prevalence is 2.4% [1]. Although the majority of individuals with BPPV are females over the age of 50, an individual's health-related quality of life is negatively affected regardless of gender or age [2]. BPPV is often associated with anxiety and depression [3]; and it may lead to falls, especially in older adults, because of its impact upon both static and dynamic postural control [4]. The primary cause of BPPV is believed to be the aging process [5]. However, traumatic brain injuries [6] and inner ear diseases [7] may also induce the signs and symptoms of BPPV, especially in individuals under the age of 50. This chapter will discuss (a) an overview of the vestibular system; (b) an overview of BPPV, including the characteristics of the nystagmus associated with each type of BPPV; (c) the methods used to evaluate each type of BPPV; and (d) the methods used to treat each type of BPPV.

Overview of the Vestibular System

The ear may be divided into an outer compartment, a middle compartment, and an inner compartment (see Figure 1) [8]. The inner ear houses the cochlea (the auditory organ designed for hearing), the labyrinth (the vestibular organ designed for balance), and cranial nerve VIII (an anatomical structure that includes both the cochlear nerve and the vestibular nerve). Together, the labyrinth and the vestibular nerve make up what is known as the peripheral vestibular system (see Figure 2) [8-9]. The labyrinth, which lies within the temporal bone, is approximately one inch in diameter [9]. It is composed of an outer bony portion that is filled with a fluid called perilymph and an inner membranous portion that is filled with a fluid called endolymph [8-9]. Three semicircular canals and two otolithic organs are housed within the labyrinth.

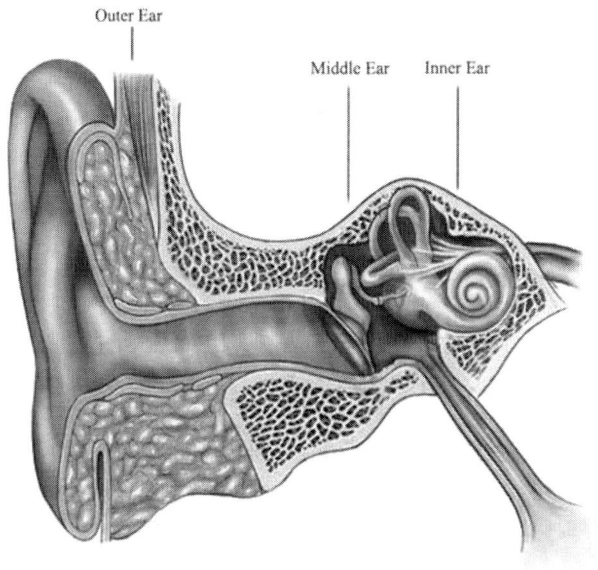

Figure 1. The Ear (image designed by Tess Tobolic).

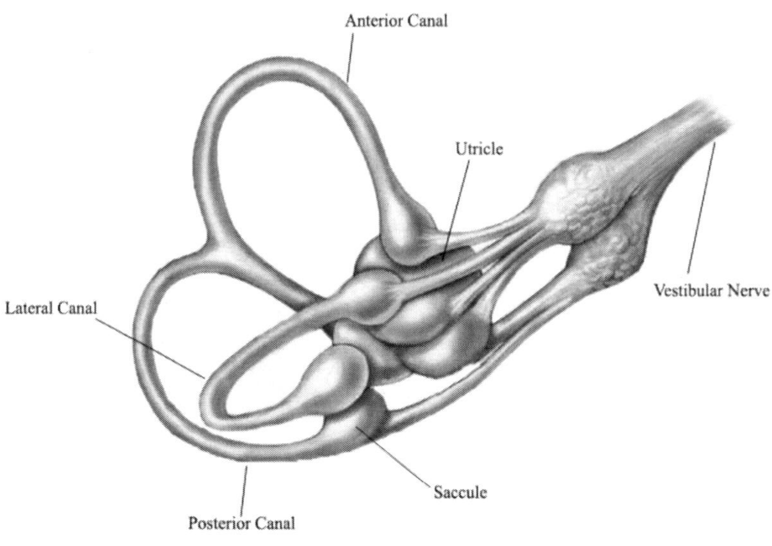

Figure 2. The Peripheral Vestibular System (image designed by Tess Tobolic).

The three semicircular canals are known as the posterior (or inferior) canal, the anterior (or superior) canal, and the lateral (or horizontal) canal [8-9]. Each semicircular canal contains an open end and a closed end [9]. At the open end, the endolymph of the semicircular canal comes into contact with the endolymph of one of the otolithic organs. At the closed end, there is a bulbous enlargement called the ampulla. Two anatomical structures are housed within each of the three ampullae, the crista (a prominent thickening located on the inferior surface of the ampulla) and the cupula (a gelatinous fluid located between the crista and the superior surface of the ampulla). Hair cells are embedded within this gelatinous fluid, and each hair cell contains several stereocilia (short, thin fibers) and one kinocilium (a long, thick fiber) [8-9]. During a rotational movement of the head, the endolymph moves in the opposite direction of the head movement. This endolymph movement compresses the cupula and causes the embedded hair cells to bend away from the endolymph. If the hair cells are bent such that the stereocilia deviate toward the kinocilium, the hair cells are said to be activated; and a depolarization of the vestibular nerve occurs. If the hair cells are bent such that the stereocilia deviate away from the kinocilium, the hair cells are said to be deactivated; and a hyperpolarization of the vestibular nerve occurs. In this way, the semicircular canals are sensitive to rotational head movements [8].

The two otolithic organs are known as the utricle and the saccule [8-9]. Two anatomical structures are housed within each of the two otolithic organs, the macula (a prominent thickening located on the inferior surface of the utricle and on the medial surface of the saccule) and the otoconia (calcium-carbonate crystals that adhere to a gelatinous fluid overlying the macula) [9]. Hair cells are embedded within this gelatinous fluid, and each hair cell contains several stereocilia (short, thin fibers) and one kinocilium (a long, thick fiber) [8-9]. During a linear movement of the head, the weight of the otoconia produces a gravitational shearing force upon the hair cells. If the hair cells are bent such that the stereocilia deviate toward the kinocilium, the hair cells are said to be activated; and a depolarization of the vestibular nerve occurs. If the hair cells are bent such that the stereocilia deviate away from the kinocilium, the hair cells are said to be deactivated; and a hyperpolarization of the vestibular nerve occurs. In this way, the otolithic organs are sensitive to linear head movements [8].

The vestibular nerve is responsible for transmitting vestibular information from the inner ear to the brain [8-9]. Four paired anatomical structures (the superior vestibular nuclei, the medial vestibular nuclei, the lateral vestibular nuclei, and the inferior vestibular nuclei) act as the primary processors of this vestibular input, and the cerebellum serves as the adaptive processor. In addition to the vestibular input, the vestibular nuclei and the cerebellum also process other sensory information such as visual input and somatosensory input. After all of this sensory input has been processed, a portion of the information travels superiorly through ascending tracts via the medial longitudinal fasciculus and the oculomotor nuclei to control the movements of the extraocular muscles. One of the primary functions of the vestibular system is to stabilize the eyes during movements of the head, and this function is accomplished through a physiological activity known as the vestibulo-ocular reflex. The remaining information travels inferiorly through descending tracts via the lateral and medial vestibulo-spinal tracts as well as the anterior horn cells and interneurons to control the movements of the skeletal muscles. The other primary function of the vestibular system is to stabilize the body during movements of the head, and this function is accomplished through a physiological activity known as the vestibulo-spinal reflex. Together, the vestibular nuclei, the ascending tracts, and the descending tracts make up what is known as the central vestibular system (see Figure 3).

Overview of BPPV

BPPV occurs when otoconia become detached from the utricle of the affected inner ear and travel into one of the semicircular canals. If the otoconia remain free floating in the endolymph of that particular semicircular canal, this condition is known as canalolithiasis [10]. If the otoconia become attached to the cupula of that particular semicircular canal, this condition is known as cupulolithiasis [11]. Because otoconia have been known to travel into all three semicircular canals, the specific types of BPPV are posterior (or inferior) canal BPPV, anterior (or superior) canal BPPV, and lateral (or horizontal) canal BPPV.

Posterior canal BPPV, the most common type of BPPV, was initially described in detail by Dix and Hallpike [12] in 1952. This type of BPPV is characterized by a spinning sensation that is elicited whenever an individual looks upward, rolls over in bed, and/or performs sit to supine transfers. The subjective complaints of vertigo are accompanied by an upbeating torsional nystagmus that demonstrates a relatively long latency, a relatively short duration, and fatigability upon repeated testing. In posterior canal BPPV, the torsional component of the nystagmus is usually more apparent than the upbeating component.

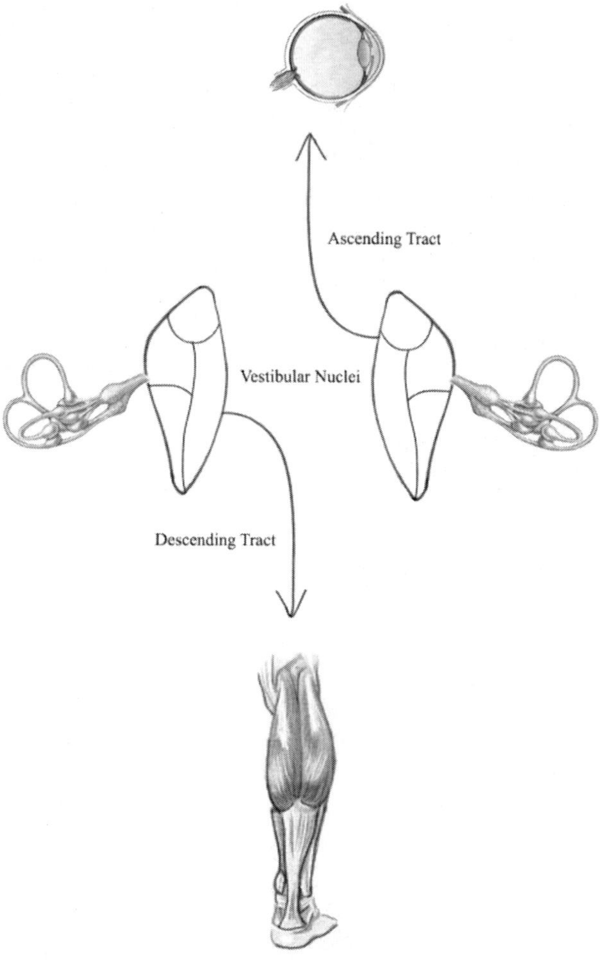

Figure 3. The Central Vestibular System (image designed by Tess Tobolic).

Anterior canal BPPV, the least common type of BPPV, was introduced by Katsarkas [13] in 1987. Like posterior canal BPPV, this type of BPPV is characterized by a spinning sensation that is elicited whenever an individual looks upward, rolls over in bed, and/or performs sit to supine transfers. Although the nystagmus that accompanies the subjective complaints of vertigo is similar to that of posterior canal BPPV in terms of its latency, duration, and fatigability, it is downbeating torsional in nature. In anterior canal BPPV, the downbeating component of the nystagmus is usually more apparent than the torsional component.

Lateral canal BPPV was introduced by McClure [14] in 1985. Although this type of BPPV is also characterized by a spinning sensation that is elicited whenever an individual rolls over in bed, vertical head movements (such as those which occur while looking upward and/or performing sit to supine transfers) seldom cause any symptoms. In lateral canal BPPV, the subjective complaints of vertigo are accompanied by a horizontal nystagmus that demonstrates a relatively short latency, a relatively long duration, and no fatigability upon repeated testing.

Evaluation Methods

A recent clinical practice guideline [15] offered a strong recommendation that the Dix-Hallpike test [12] be used to evaluate individuals with suspected cases of posterior canal BPPV. In individual studies, this test was shown to have a sensitivity of 82% and a specificity of 71% [16] as well as a positive predictive value of 83% and a negative predictive value of 52% [17]. In addition, a recent critically appraised topic [18] reported that the Dix-Hallpike test has a sensitivity of approximately 79%, a specificity of approximately 75%, a positive predictive value of approximately 96%, and a negative predictive value of approximately 33%. The Dix-Hallpike test is performed in a series of four steps: (a) the individual assumes a long-sitting position with the head rotated 45 degrees to the right (see Figure 4); (b) the individual is moved into a supine position with the head slightly extended off the end of the treatment table (see Figure 5); (c) the individual assumes a long-sitting position with the head rotated 45 degrees to the left; and (d) the individual is moved into a supine position with the head slightly extended off the end of the treatment table.

If the individual demonstrates upbeating right torsional nystagmus at the conclusion of the second step, the diagnosis is considered to be right-sided posterior canal BPPV. If the individual demonstrates upbeating left torsional nystagmus at the conclusion of the fourth step, the diagnosis is considered to be left-sided posterior canal BPPV. Canalolithiasis of the posterior semicircular canal is characterized by a relatively short duration of the elicited nystagmus, and cupulolithiasis of the posterior semicircular canal is characterized by a relatively long duration of the elicited nystagmus.

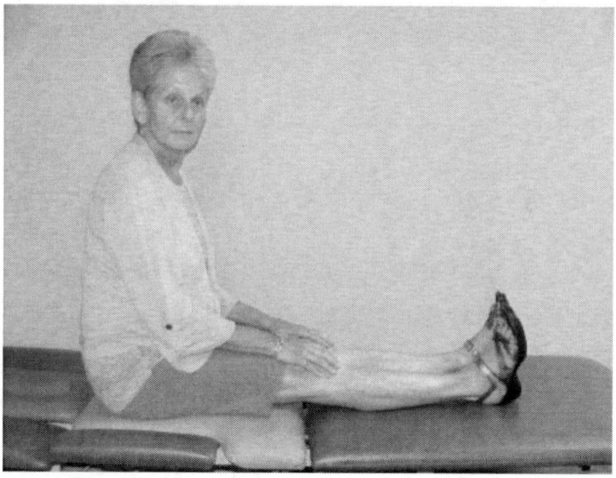

Figure 4. Step one of the Dix-Hallpike test.

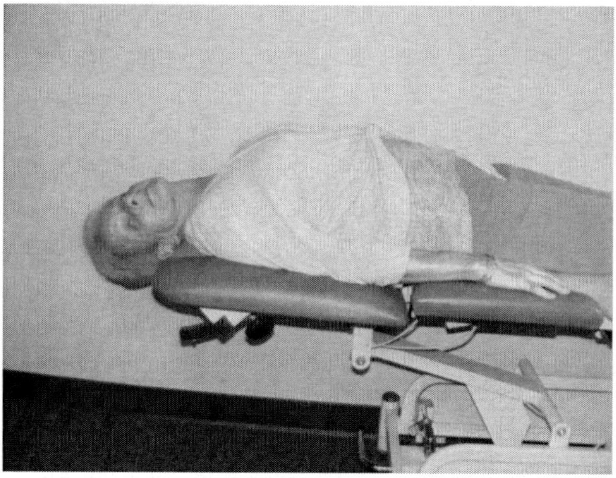

Figure 5. Step two of the Dix-Hallpike test.

Although anterior canal BPPV is sometimes detected when the Dix-Hallpike test is performed, this type of BPPV is more effectively diagnosed with the head hanging test [19]. The head hanging test is performed in a series of two steps: (a) the individual assumes a long-sitting position with the head in neutral (see Figure 6); and (b) the individual is moved into a supine position with the head completely extended off the end of the treatment table (see Figure 7). If the individual demonstrates downbeating right torsional nystagmus at the conclusion of the second step, the diagnosis is considered to be right-sided anterior canal BPPV. If the individual demonstrates downbeating left torsional nystagmus at the conclusion of the second step, the diagnosis is considered to be left-sided anterior canal BPPV. Canalolithiasis of the anterior semicircular canal is characterized by a relatively short duration of the elicited nystagmus, and cupulolithiasis of the anterior semicircular canal is characterized by a relatively long duration of the elicited nystagmus.

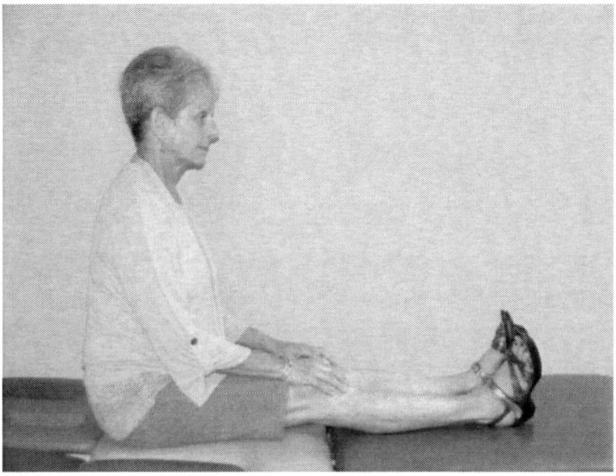

Figure 6. Step one of the head hanging test.

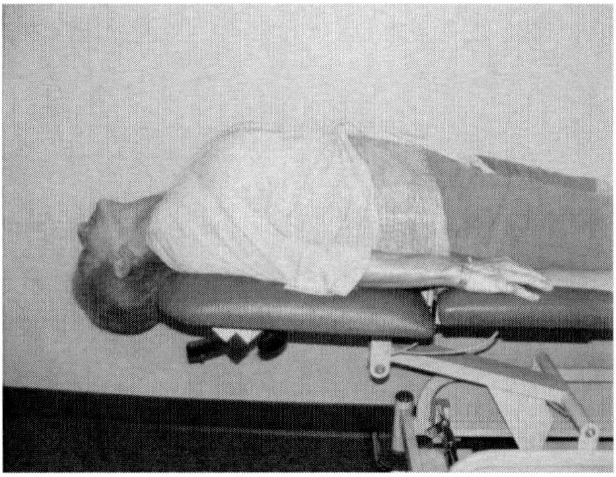

Figure 7. Step two of the head hanging test.

A recent clinical practice guideline [15] offered a positive recommendation that the head roll test [20] be used to evaluate individuals with suspected cases of lateral canal BPPV. The head roll test is performed in a series of four steps: (a) the individual assumes a supine position, usually with the head flexed 20 to 30 degrees (see Figure 8); (b) the individual's head is rotated 45 degrees to the right (see Figure 9); (c) the individual assumes a supine position, usually with the head flexed 20 to 30 degrees; and (d) the individual's head is rotated 45 degrees to the left.

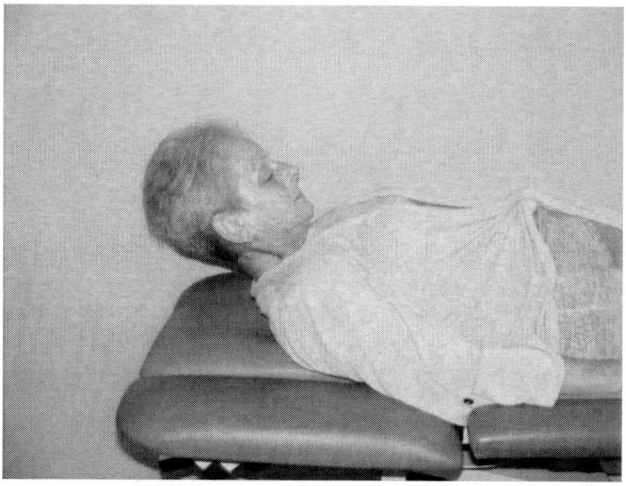

Figure 8. Step one of the head roll test.

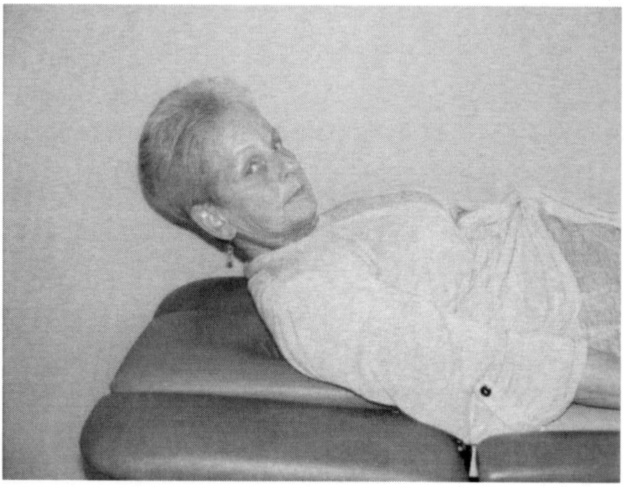

Figure 9. Step two of the head roll test.

The direction and intensity of the elicited nystagmus at the conclusion of steps two and four are then compared. If the individual demonstrates right-beating nystagmus when the head is rotated to the right and left-beating nystagmus when the head is rotated to the left, the individual is diagnosed with geotropic nystagmus [14]. The presence of free-floating otoconia in the posterior arm of the lateral semicircular canal (canalolithisis) is believed to be the cause of this type of nystagmus. If the individual demonstrates left-beating nystagmus when the head is rotated to the right and right-beating nystagmus when the head is rotated to the left, the individual is diagnosed with apogeotropic nystagmus [21]. The presence of free-floating otoconia in the anterior arm of the lateral semicircular canal (canalolithiasis) [22] or the attachment of otoconia to the cupula in the lateral semicircular canal (cupulolithiasis) [21] is believed to be the cause of this type of nystagmus. In addition, it has been hypothesized that the involved ear is the one towards which the greatest intensity of nystagmus is directed when the head roll test is performed [20-21].

Treatment Methods

Several treatment methods have been successfully applied to individuals with each type of BPPV. Therefore, this section is divided into (a) interventions for posterior canal BPPV, (b) interventions for anterior canal BPPV, and (c) interventions for lateral canal BPPV.

Posterior Canal BPPV Interventions

If an individual is diagnosed with canalolithiasis of the posterior semicircular canal, the most popular treatment approach is the Epley canalith repositioning procedure, an intervention that was created by Epley [23] in 1992. The original Epley canalith repositioning procedure is performed in a series of six steps: (a) if the diagnosis is right-sided posterior canal BPPV, the individual assumes a long-sitting position with the head rotated 45 degrees to the right (see Figure 10); (b) the individual is moved into a supine position with the head slightly extended off the end of the treatment table (see Figure 11); (c) once the elicited nystagmus has subsided, the individual's head is rotated 90 degrees to the left (see Figure 12); (d) once the elicited nystagmus has subsided, the individual is moved into a left side-lying position (see Figure 13); (e) once the elicited nystagmus has subsided, the individual is moved into a sitting position (see Figure 14); and (f) once the elicited nystagmus has subsided, the individual's head is moved so that it is in 0 degrees of rotation and approximately 20 degrees of flexion (see Figure 15).

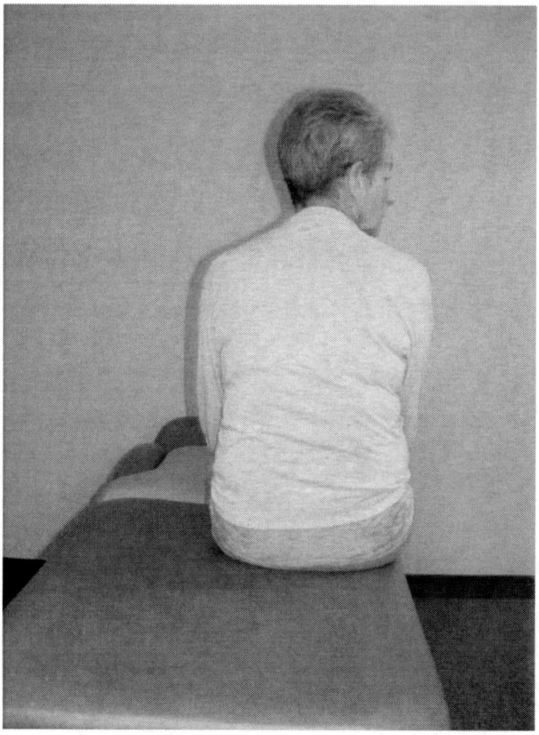

Figure 10. Step one of the Epley canalith repositioning procedure.

This sequence is repeated until nystagmus is no longer elicited. If the diagnosis is left-sided posterior canal BPPV, the individual assumes a long-sitting position with the head rotated 45 degrees to the left during step one; and the subsequent steps are performed in mirror image to the right-sided intervention.

During the initial study, approximately 90% of the participants experienced a complete resolution of their vertigo and nystagmus after a single treatment session. Since the time of this initial investigation, four case series [24-27] and three randomized controlled trials [28-30] have examined the effectiveness of the original Epley canalith repositioning procedure.

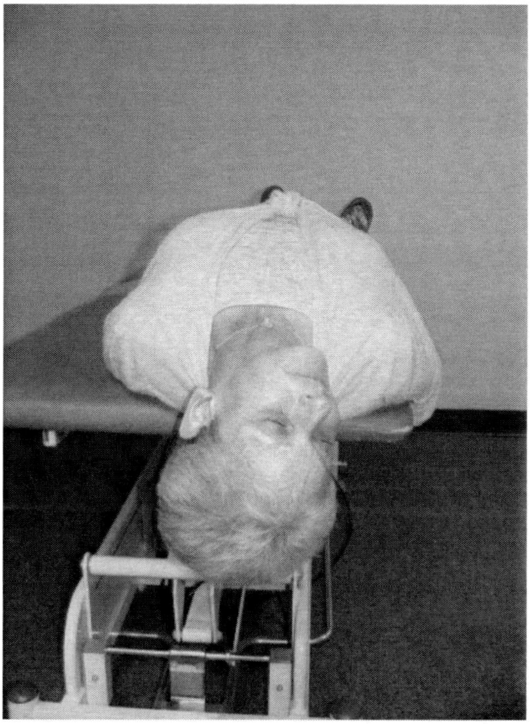

Figure 11. Step two of the Epley canalith repositioning procedure.

During the four case series, 56% [27] to 87% [26] of the participants experienced a complete resolution of their vertigo and nystagmus after a single treatment session. During the three randomized controlled trials, the one-treatment success rate of the Epley procedure was 67% [28] to 89% [29] while the one-treatment success rate of a sham maneuver was 10% [30] to 38% [28]. Although each of these studies investigated the original version of the Epley canalith repositioning procedure, it should be noted that most clinicians currently use a modification of the original maneuver. In addition to the four case series and the three randomized controlled trials just described, two recent clinical practice guidelines [15,31] have analyzed the effectiveness of the original and/or the modified Epley procedure. One clinical practice guideline [15] offered a positive recommendation that individuals with posterior canal BPPV be treated with the Epley canalith repositioning procedure. The other clinical practice guideline [31] offered a level A recommendation that the Epley canalith repositioning procedure is effective when treating individuals with posterior canal BPPV.

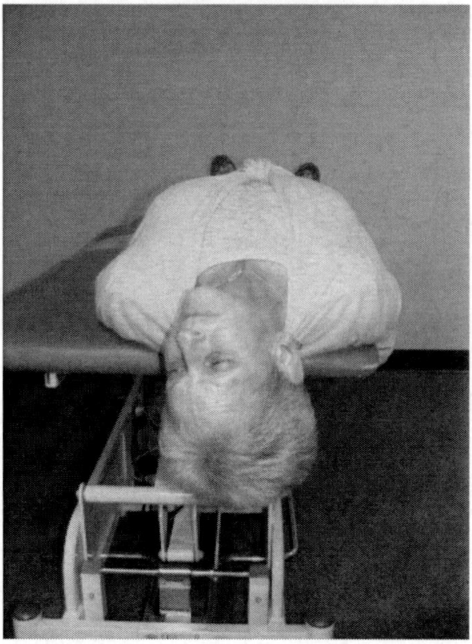

Figure 12. Step three of the Epley canalith repositioning procedure.

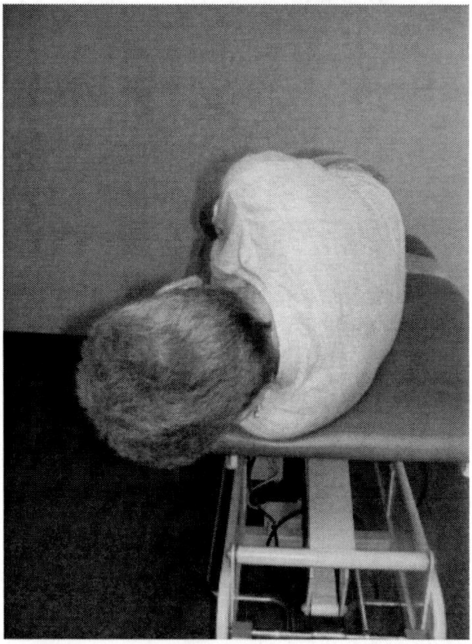

Figure 13. Step four of the Epley canalith repositioning procedure.

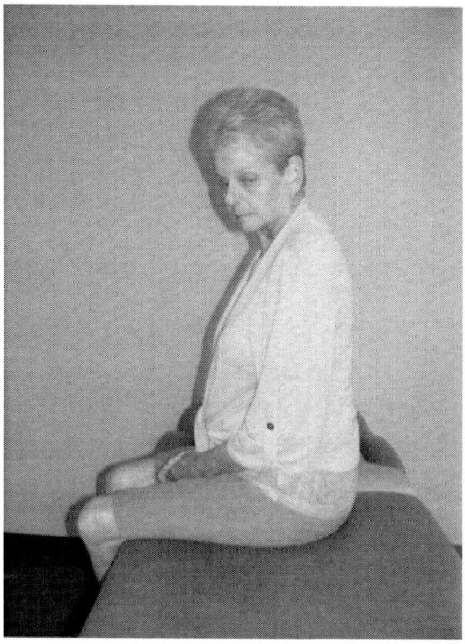

Figure 14. Step five of the Epley canalith repositioning procedure.

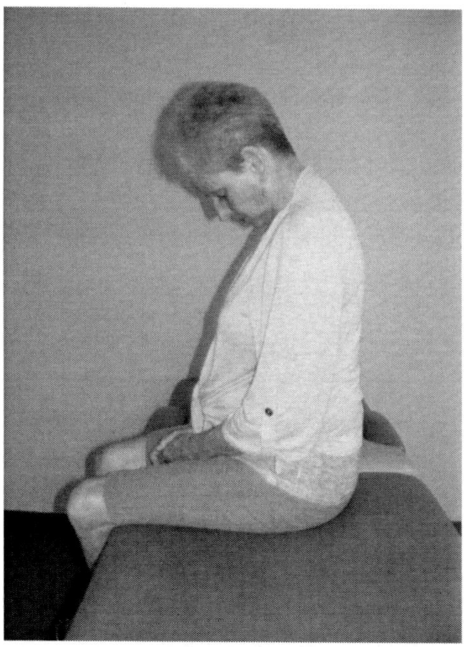

Figure 15. Step six of the Epley canalith repositioning procedure.

If an individual is diagnosed with cupulolithiasis of the posterior semicircular canal, the most popular treatment approach is the Semont liberatory maneuver, an intervention that was created by Semont, Freyss, and Vitte [32] in 1988. The Semont liberatory maneuver is performed in a series of three steps: (a) if the diagnosis is right-sided posterior canal BPPV, the individual assumes a sitting position with the head rotated 45 degrees to the left (see Figure 16); (b) the individual is moved into a right side-lying position and once the elicited nystagmus has subsided, the individual remains in this position for two to three minutes (see Figure 17); and (c) the individual is moved up into a sitting position and down into a left side-lying position in one continuous motion and once the elicited nystagmus has subsided, the individual remains in this position for five minutes (see Figure 18). If the diagnosis is left-sided posterior canal BPPV, the individual assumes a sitting position with the head rotated 45 degrees to the right during step one; and the subsequent steps are performed in mirror image to the right-sided intervention. During the initial study, approximately 84% of the participants experienced a complete resolution of their vertigo and nystagmus after a single treatment session. Since the time of this initial investigation, five case series [33-37] and one randomized controlled trial [38] have examined the effectiveness of the Semont liberatory maneuver. During the five case series, 35% [34] to 81% [37] of the participants experienced a complete resolution of their vertigo and nystagmus after a single treatment session. During the randomized controlled trial [38], the one-treatment success rate of the Semont maneuver was 87% while the one-treatment success rate of a sham procedure was 0%. In addition to the five case series and the one randomized controlled trial just described, two recent clinical practice guidelines [15,31] have analyzed the effectiveness of the Semont maneuver. One clinical practice guideline [15] offered a positive recommendation that individuals with posterior canal BPPV be treated with the Semont liberatory maneuver. The other clinical practice guideline [31] offered a level C recommendation that the Semont liberatory maneuver is effective when treating individuals with posterior canal BPPV.

The Epley canalith repositioning procedure [23] and the Semont liberatory maneuver [32] are each administered by a clinician. In addition to these two clinician-administered interventions, the Brandt-Daroff exercise [39] is a posterior canal BPPV activity that may be self-administered at home. This exercise was created by Brandt and Daroff in 1980, and it is performed in a series of four steps: (a) while sitting on the edge of a bed, the individual turns the head to the left and lies down on the right side; (b) after 30 seconds have elapsed, the individual returns to a seated position; (c) after 30 seconds have elapsed, the individual turns the head to the right and lies down on the left side; and (d) after 30 seconds have elapsed, the individual returns to a seated position. This sequence is repeated until vertigo is no longer elicited, and the exercise is performed every three hours during the day until the individual experiences two consecutive symptom-free days.

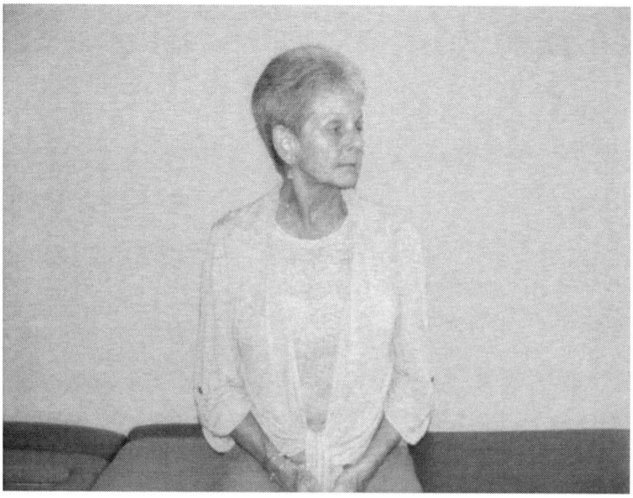

Figure 16. Step one of the Semont liberatory maneuver.

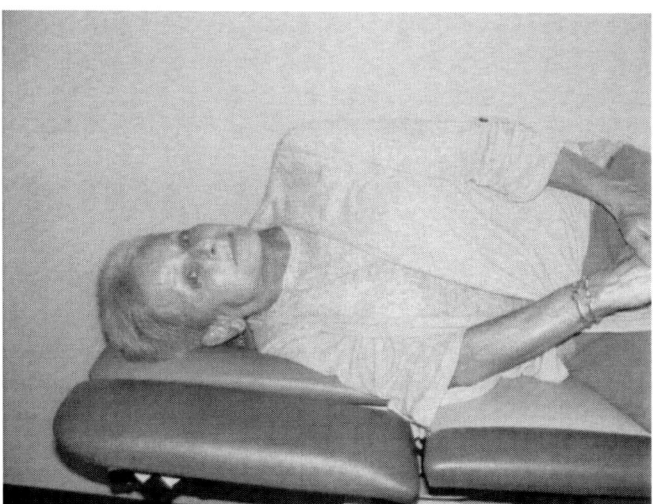

Figure 17. Step two of the Semont liberatory maneuver.

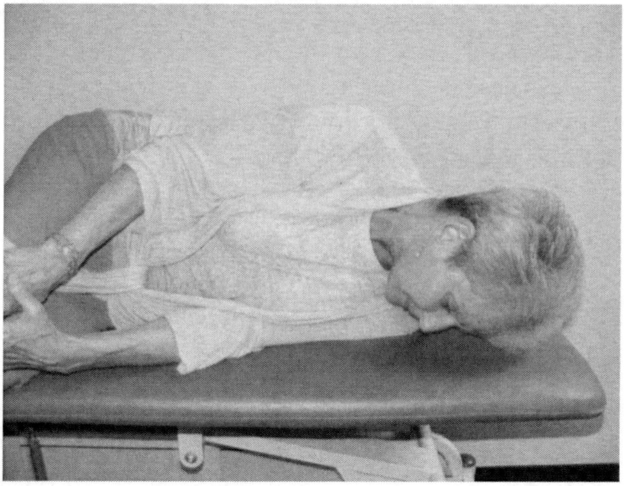

Figure 18. Step three of the Semont liberatory maneuver.

During the initial study, approximately 99% of the participants experienced a complete resolution of their vertigo and nystagmus within 3 to 14 days of beginning this exercise. Despite this high rate of success, one recent clinical practice guideline [15] stated that when considering the use of the Brandt-Daroff exercise as the initial treatment option for posterior canal BPPV, the quality of the supporting evidence is questionable and/or the evidence obtained from high-quality investigations is unclear. In addition, another recent clinical practice guideline [31] stated that when considering the effectiveness of a self-administered maneuver (such as the Brandt-Daroff exercise) for treating individuals with posterior canal BPPV, the intervention is unproven and/or the evidence is unclear.

Anterior Canal BPPV Interventions

Historically, individuals diagnosed with anterior canal BPPV were treated with the use of a posterior canal BPPV intervention such as the Epley canalith repositioning procedure, the Semont liberatory maneuver, and/or the Brandt-Daroff exercise. These posterior canal BPPV interventions, when used in "reverse", were also commonly used. Then, in 2014, a systematic review [40] revealed four interventions that were specifically developed for the treatment of anterior canal BPPV.

The first intervention, created by Kim, Shin, and Chung [41] in 2005, is performed in a series of five steps: (a) if the diagnosis is right-sided anterior canal BPPV, the individual assumes a long-sitting position with the head rotated 45 degrees to the left; (b) the individual is moved into a supine position with the head extended 45 degrees off the end of the treatment table; (c) after two minutes have elapsed, the individual's head is flexed 45 degrees until it is in a neutral position with respect to flexion and extension; (d) after one minute has elapsed, the individual is moved into a long-sitting position with the head flexed 30 degrees; and (e) the individual's head is rotated 45 degrees to the right until it is in a neutral position with respect to rotation. If the diagnosis is left-sided anterior canal BPPV, the individual assumes a long-sitting position with the head rotated 45 degrees to the right during step one; and the subsequent steps are performed in mirror image to the right-sided intervention. During the initial study, approximately 47% of the participants experienced a complete resolution of their vertigo and nystagmus after a single treatment session.

The second intervention, created by Yacovino, Hain, and Gualtieri [42] in 2009, is performed in a series of five steps: (a) the individual assumes a long-sitting position with the head in neutral; (b) the individual is moved into a supine position with the head extended at least 30 degrees off the end of the treatment table; (c) after 30 seconds have elapsed, the individual's head is completely flexed; (d) after 30 seconds have elapsed, the individual is moved into a long-sitting position with the head in neutral, and (e) the individual remains in this final position for 30 seconds. During the initial study, approximately 85% of the participants experienced a complete resolution of their vertigo and nystagmus after a single treatment session.

The third intervention, created by Korres, Riga, Sandris, Danielides, and Sismanis [43] in 2010, is performed in a series of five steps: (a) if the diagnosis is right-sided anterior canal BPPV, the individual assumes a long-sitting position with the head rotated 45 degrees to the right; (b) the individual is moved into a supine position with the head completely extended off the end of the treatment table; (c) after one minute has elapsed, the individual's head is rotated 90 degrees to the left; (d) after one minute has elapsed, the individual is moved into a long-sitting position with the head in a neutral position with respect to flexion and extension, and (e) the individual remains in this final position for one to two minutes. If the diagnosis is left-sided anterior canal BPPV, the individual assumes a long-sitting position with the head rotated 45 degrees to the left during step one; and the subsequent steps are performed in mirror image to the right-sided intervention. During the initial study, approximately 60% of the participants experienced a complete resolution of their vertigo and nystagmus after a single treatment session.

The fourth intervention, created by Casani, Cerchiai, Dallan, and Sellari-Franceschini [44] in 2011, is performed in a series of four steps: (a) the individual assumes a long-sitting position with the head in neutral; (b) the individual is moved into a supine position with the head completely extended off the end of the treatment table; (c) after three minutes have elapsed, the individual's head is completely flexed; and (d) after three minutes have elapsed, the individual is moved into a long-sitting position with the head in neutral. This sequence is then repeated one more time. During the initial study, approximately 44% of the participants experienced a complete resolution of their vertigo and nystagmus after a single treatment session.

Lateral Canal BPPV Interventions

In 2012, a systematic review [45] revealed three effective interventions for treating the geotropic variant of lateral canal BPPV and two potential interventions for treating the apogeotropic variant of lateral canal BPPV. The geotropic interventions included the Gufoni maneuver, the 270-degree roll technique, and prolonged position. The apogeotropic interventions included the modified Semont maneuver and the head shaking technique. The Gufoni maneuver, the 270-degree roll technique, the modified Semont maneuver, and the head shaking technique are each administered by a clinician. Prolonged position, on the other hand, is a lateral canal BPPV activity that may be self-administered at home.

The Gufoni maneuver, initially described in detail by Asprella-Libonati [46] in 2005, is performed in a series of four steps: (a) the individual assumes a sitting position with the head in neutral (see Figure 19); (b) if the diagnosis is right-sided lateral canal BPPV, the individual is moved into a left side-lying position (see Figure 20); (c) the individual's head is rotated 45 degrees to the left (see Figure 21); and (d) the individual remains in this final position for two to three minutes. If the diagnosis is left-sided lateral canal BPPV, the individual is moved into a right-sidelying position during step two; and the subsequent step is performed in mirror image to the right-sided intervention. In the 2012 systematic review [45], the Gufoni maneuver demonstrated the best short-term success rate as approximately 86% of the participants experienced a complete resolution of their vertigo and nystagmus after one treatment [47].

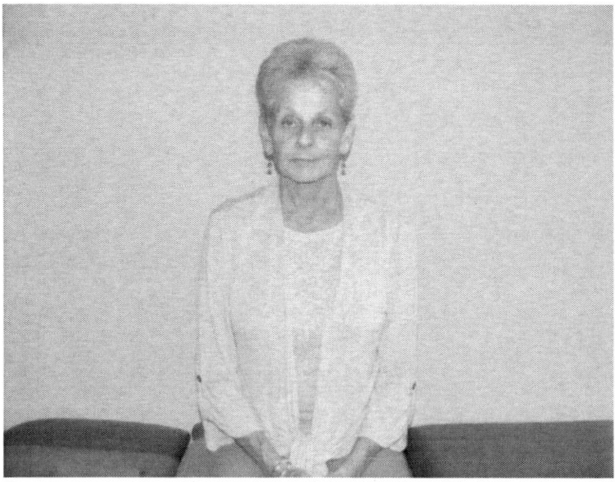

Figure 19. Step one of the Gufoni maneuver.

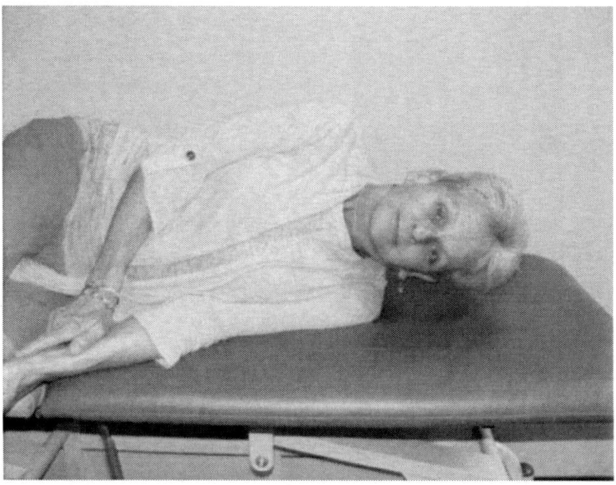

Figure 20. Step two of the Gufoni maneuver.

The 270-degree roll technique, created by Lempert [48] in 1994, is performed in a series of five steps: (a) the individual assumes a supine position with the head in neutral (see Figure 22); (b) if the diagnosis is right-sided lateral canal BPPV, the individual is moved into a left side-lying position (see Figure 23); (c) after 30 seconds have elapsed, the individual is moved into a prone position (see Figure 24); (d) after 30 seconds have elapsed, the individual is moved into a right side-lying position (see Figure 25); and (e) the individual remains in this final position for 30 seconds.

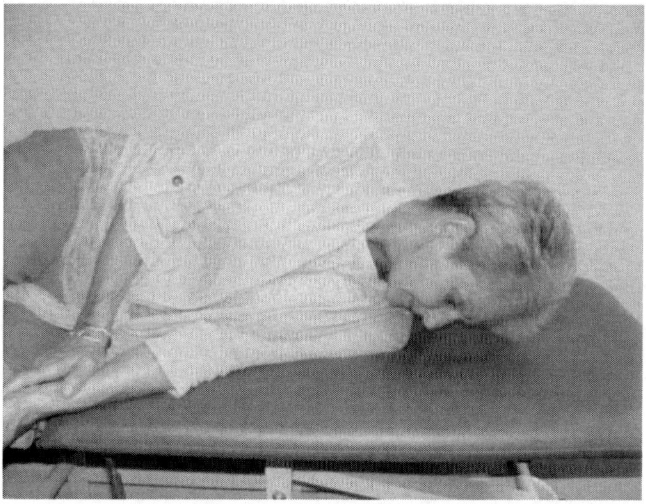

Figure 21. Step three of the Gufoni maneuver.

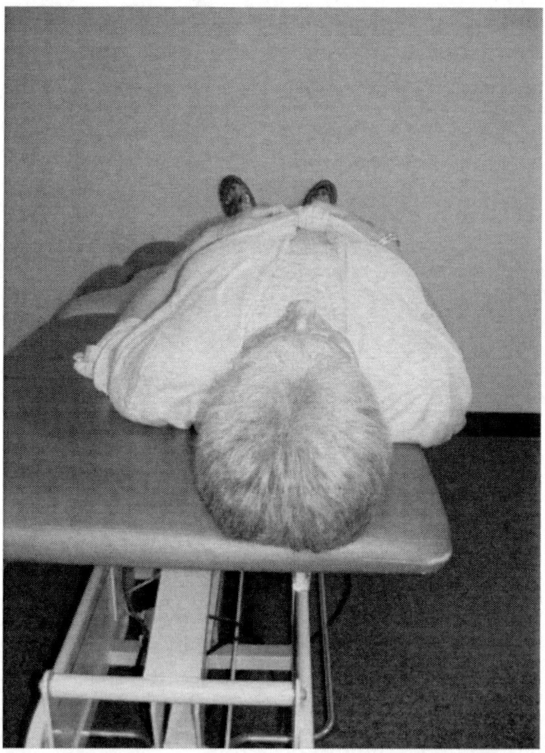

Figure 22. Step one of the 270-degree roll technique.

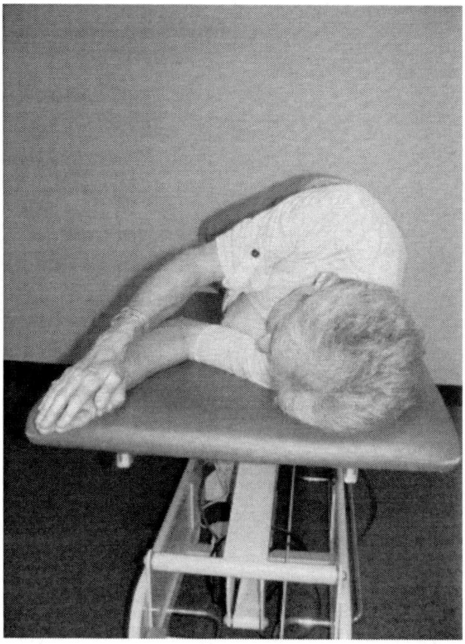

Figure 23. Step two of the 270-degree roll technique.

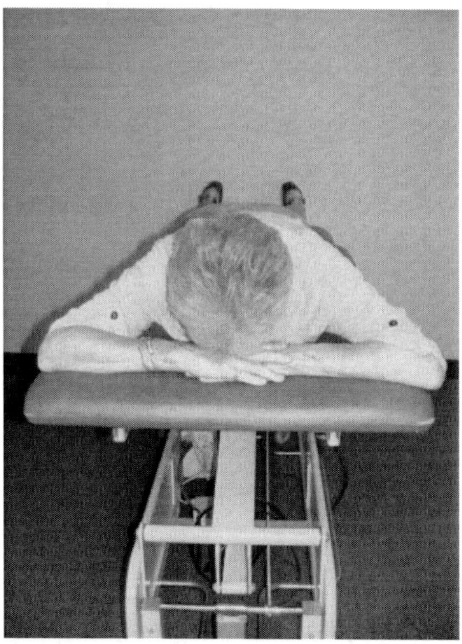

Figure 24. Step three of the 270-degree roll technique.

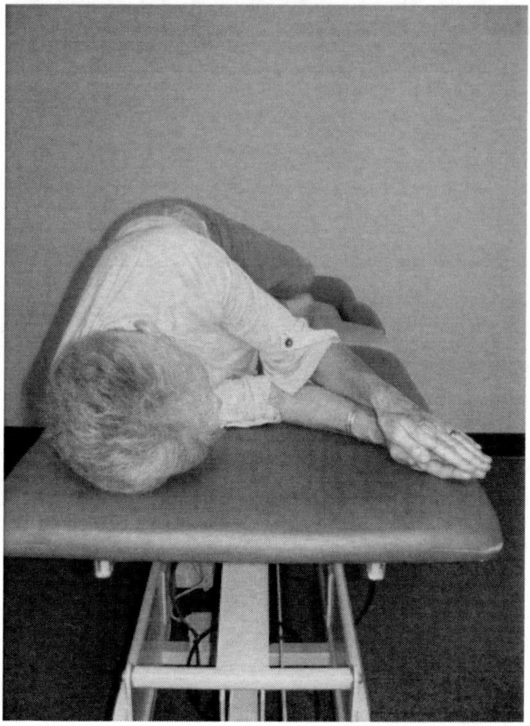

Figure 25. Step four of the 270-degree roll technique.

If the diagnosis is left-sided lateral canal BPPV, the individual is moved into a right side-lying position during step two; and the subsequent steps are performed in mirror image to the right-sided intervention. In the 2012 systematic review [45], the 270-degree roll technique demonstrated the best long-term success rate as approximately 97% of the participants experienced a complete resolution of their vertigo and nystagmus after one month [49].

Prolonged position, created by Vannucchi, Giannoni, and Pagnini [50] in 1997, is performed in a series of three steps: (a) the individual assumes a supine position with the head in neutral; (b) if the diagnosis is right-sided lateral canal BPPV, the individual rolls over onto the left side; and (c) the individual remains in this final position for approximately 12 hours. If the diagnosis is left-sided lateral canal BPPV, the individual rolls over onto the right side during step two.

The modified Semont maneuver, created by Casani, Vannucci, Fattori, and Berrettini [51] in 2002, is performed in a series of four steps: (a) the individual assumes a sitting position with the head in neutral; (b) if the diagnosis is right-sided lateral canal BPPV, the individual is moved into a right side-lying position; (c) the individual's head is rotated 45 degrees to the right; and (d) the individual remains in this final position for two to three minutes. If the diagnosis is left-sided lateral canal BPPV, the individual is moved into a left-sidelying position during step two; and the subsequent step is performed in mirror image to the right-sided intervention.

In the 2012 systematic review [45], the modified Semont maneuver demonstrated a 13% one-treatment success rate in one of the included studies [52] and a 44% one-treatment success rate in the other included study [51].

The head shaking technique, created by Oh et al. [52] in 2009, is performed in a series of three steps: (a) the individual assumes a sitting position with the head flexed 30 degrees; (b) the individual's head is quickly rotated back and forth for 15 seconds; and (c) the patient remains in a sitting position with the head flexed 30 degrees for approximately 30 minutes. In the 2012 systematic review [45], the head shaking technique demonstrated a 33% one-treatment success rate in the only included study [52] in which it was investigated.

Conclusion

BPPV, one of the most common disorders of the vestibular system, occurs when otoconia become detached from the utricle of the affected inner ear and travel into one of the semicircular canals. Because otoconia have been known to travel into all three semicircular canals, the specific types of BPPV are posterior (or inferior) canal BPPV, anterior (or superior) canal BPPV, and lateral (or horizontal) canal BPPV. Posterior canal BPPV is most effectively diagnosed with the Dix-Hallpike test. If an individual is diagnosed with canalolithiasis of the posterior semicircular canal, the most popular treatment approach is the Epley canalith repositioning procedure; and if an individual is diagnosed with cupulolithiasis of the posterior semicircular canal, the most popular treatment approach is the Semont liberatory maneuver. The Epley procedure and the Semont maneuver are each administered by a clinician. In addition to these two clinician-administered interventions, the Brandt-Daroff exercise is a posterior canal BPPV activity that may be self-administered at home. Anterior canal BPPV is most effectively diagnosed with the head hanging test. A 2014 systematic review revealed four interventions that were specifically developed for the treatment of anterior canal BPPV. Lateral canal

BPPV is most effectively diagnosed with the head roll test. A 2012 systematic review revealed three effective interventions for treating the geotropic variant of lateral canal BPPV and two potential interventions for treating the apogeotropic variant of lateral canal BPPV.

References

[1] VonBrevern, M., Radtke, A., Lezius, F., Feldmann, M., Ziese, T., Lempert, T. & Neuhauser, H. (2007). Epidemiology of benign paroxysmal positional vertigo: A population based study. *Journal of Neurology, Neurosurgery, and Psychiatry*, *78*, 710-715.

[2] Roberts, R. A., Abrams, H., Sembach, M. K., Lister, J. J., Gans, R. E. & Chisholm, T. H. (2009). Utility measures of health-related quality of life in patients treated for benign paroxysmal positional vertigo. *Ear and Hearing*, *30*, 369-376.

[3] Pollak, L., Segal, P., Stryjer, R. & Stern, H. G. (2012). Beliefs and emotional reactions in patients with benign paroxysmal positional vertigo: A longitudinal study. *American Journal of Otolaryngology*, *33*, 221-225.

[4] Gananca, F. F., Gazzola, J. M., Gananca, C. F., Caovilla, H. H., Gananca, M. M. & Cruz, O. L. M. (2010). Elderly falls associated with benign paroxysmal positional vertigo. *Brazilian Journal of Otorhinolaryngology*, *76*, 113-120.

[5] Faralli, M., Ricci, G., Molini, E., Bressi, T., Simoncelli, C. & Frenguelli, A. (2006). Paroxysmal positional vertigo: The role of age as a prognostic factor. *Acta Otorhinolaryngologica Italica*, *26*, 25-31.

[6] Ahn, S. K., Jeon, S. Y., Kim, J. P., Park, J. J., Hur, D. G., Kim, D. W.,... . Kim, J. Y. (2011). Clinical characteristics and treatment of benign paroxysmal positional vertigo after traumatic brain injury. *Journal of Trauma*, *70*, 442-446.

[7] Lee, N. H., Ban, J. H., Lee, K. C. & Kim, S. M. (2010). Benign paroxysmal positional vertigo secondary to inner ear disease. *Otolaryngology: Head and Neck Surgery*, *143*, 413-417.

[8] Hain, T. C. & Helminski, J. O. (2007). Anatomy and physiology of the normal vestibular system. In S. J. Herdman (Ed.), Vestibular rehabilitation (3rd ed., 2-18). Philadelphia, PA: F. A. Davis Company.

[9] Crutchfield, C. A. & Barnes, M. R. (1993). Anatomy and physiology of the vestibular system. In C. A. Crutchfield & M. R. Barnes (Eds.), Motor control and motor learning in rehabilitation (277-312). Atlanta, GA: Stokesville Publishing Company.

[10] Hall, S. F., Ruby, R. R. F. & McClure, J. A. (1979). The mechanics of benign paroxysmal vertigo. *Journal of Otolaryngology*, *8*, 151-158.

[11] Schuknecht, H. F. (1969). Cupulolithiasis. *Archives of Otolaryngology*, *90*, 765-778.

[12] Dix, M. R. & Hallpike, C. S. (1952). The pathology, symptomatology and diagnosis of certain common disorders of the vestibular system. *Proceedings of the Royal Society of Medicine*, *45*, 341-354.

[13] Katsarkas, A. (1987). Nystagmus of paroxysmal positional vertigo: Some new insights. *Annals of Otology, Rhinology, and Laryngology*, *96*, 305-308.

[14] McClure, J. A. (1985). Horizontal canal BPV. *Journal of Otolaryngology*, *14*, 30-35.

[15] Bhattacharyya, N., Baugh, R. F., Orvidas, L., Barrs, D., Bronston, L. J., Cass, S., Haidari, J. (2008). Clinical practice guideline: Benign paroxysmal positional vertigo. *Otolaryngology: Head and Neck Surgery*, *139*, S47-S81.

[16] Lopez-Escamez, J. A., Lopez-Nevot, A., Gamiz, M. J., Moreno, P. M., Bracero, F., Castillo, J. L. & Salinero, J. (2000). Diagnosis of common causes of vertigo using a structured clinical history. *Acta Otorrinolaringologica Espanola*, *51*, 25-30.

[17] Hanley, K. & O'Dowd, T. (2002). Symptoms of vertigo in general practice: A prospective study of diagnosis. *British Journal of General Practice*, *52*, 809-812.

[18] Halker, R. B., Barrs, D. M., Wellik, K. E., Wingerchuk, D. M. & Demaerschalk, B. M. (2008). Establishing a diagnosis of benign paroxysmal positional vertigo through the Dix-Hallpike and side-lying maneuvers: A critically appraised topic. *Neurologist*, *14*, 201-204.

[19] Bertholon, P., Bronstein, A. M., Davies, R. A., Rudge, P. & Thilo, K. V. (2002). Positional down beating nystagmus in 50 patients: Cerebellar disorders and possible anterior semicircular canalithiasis. *Journal of Neurology, Neurosurgery, and Psychiatry*, *72*, 366-372.

[20] Pagnini, P., Nuti, D. & Vannucchi, P. (1989). Benign paroxysmal vertigo of the horizontal canal. *ORL: Journal for Oto-Rhino-Laryngology and its Related Specialties*, *51*, 161-170.

[21] Baloh, R. W., Yue, Q., Jacobson, K. M. & Honrubia, V. (1995). Persistent direction-changing positional nystagmus: Another variant of benign positional nystagmus? *Neurology*, *45*, 1297-1301.

[22] Nuti, D., Vannucchi, P. & Pagnini, P. (1996). Benign paroxysmal positional vertigo of the horizontal canal: A form of canalolithiasis with variable clinical features. *Journal of Vestibular Research*, *6*, 173-184.

[23] Epley, J. M. (1992). The canalith repositioning procedure: For treatment of benign paroxysmal positional vertigo. *Otolaryngology: Head and Neck Surgery*, *107*, 399-404.

[24] Jose, P., Rupa, V. & Job, A. (2000). Successful management of benign paroxysmal positional vertigo with the Epley manoeuvre. *Indian Journal of Otolaryngology and Head and Neck Surgery*, *52*, 49-53.

[25] Mujeeb, M. & Khan, N. U. H. (2000). Epley's manoeuvre: Treatment of choice for benign paroxysmal positional vertigo. *Journal of Laryngology and Otology*, *114*, 844-847.

[26] Nunez, R. A., Cass, S. P. & Furman, J. M. (2000). Short- and long-term outcomes of canalith repositioning for benign paroxysmal positional vertigo. *Otolaryngology: Head and Neck Surgery*, *122*, 647-652.

[27] Smouha, E. E. (1997). Time course of recovery after Epley maneuvers for benign paroxysmal positional vertigo. *Laryngoscope*, *107*, 187-191.

[28] Froehling, D. A., Bowen, J. M., Mohr, D. N., Brey, R. H., Beatty, C. W., Wollan, P. C. & Silverstein, M. D. (2000). The canalith repositioning procedure for the treatment of benign paroxysmal positional vertigo: A randomized controlled trial. *Mayo Clinic Proceedings*, *75*, 695-700.

[29] Lynn, S., Pool, A., Rose, D., Brey, R. & Suman, V. (1995). Randomized trial of the canalith repositioning procedure. *Otolaryngology: Head and Neck Surgery*, *113*, 712-720.

[30] VonBrevern, M., Seelig, T., Radtke, A., Tiel-Wilck, K., Neuhauser, H. & Lempert, T. (2006). Short-term efficacy of Epley's manoeuvre: A double-blind randomised trial. *Journal of Neurology, Neurosurgery, and Psychiatry*, *77*, 980-982.

[31] Fife, T. D., Iverson, D. J., Lempert, T., Furman, J. M., Baloh, R. W., Tusa, R. J., Gronseth, G. S. (2008). Practice parameter: Therapies for benign paroxysmal positional vertigo (an evidence-based review). *Neurology*, *70*, 2067-2074.

[32] Semont, A., Freyss, G. & Vitte, E. (1988). Curing the BPPV with a liberatory maneuver. *Advances in Oto-Rhino-Laryngology*, *42*, 290-293.

[33] Brocchetti, F., Garaventa, G., Ameli, F., Baricalla, F., Chiarlone, M., Peirano, M., Fibbi, A. (2003). Effect of repetition of Semont's

manoeuvre on benign paroxysmal positional vertigo of posterior semicircular canal. *Acta Otorhinolaryngologica Italica*, *23*, 428-435.

[34] Kollen, L., Bjerlemo, B. & Moller, C. (2006). Evaluation of treatment in benign paroxysmal positional vertigo (BPPV). *Advances in Physiotherapy*, *8*, 106-115.

[35] Levrat, E., VanMelle, G., Monnier, P. & Maire, R. (2003). Efficacy of the Semont maneuver in benign paroxysmal positional vertigo. *Archives of Otolaryngology: Head and Neck Surgery*, *129*, 629-633.

[36] Serafini, G., Palmieri, A. M. R. & Simoncelli, C. (1996). Benign paroxysmal positional vertigo of posterior semicircular canal: Results in 160 cases treated with Semont's maneuver. *Annals of Otology, Rhinology, and Laryngology*, *105*, 770-775.

[37] Soto-Varela, A., Rossi-Izquierdo, M., Martinez-Capoccioni, G., Labella-Caballero, T. & Santos-Perez, S. (2012). Benign paroxysmal positional vertigo of the posterior semicircular canal: Efficacy of Santiago treatment protocol, long-term follow up and analysis of recurrence. *Journal of Laryngology and Otology*, *126*, 363-371.

[38] Mandala, M., Santoro, G. P., Libonati, G. A., Casani, A. P., Faralli, M., Giannoni, B., . . . Nuti, D. (2012). Double-blind randomized trial on short-term efficacy of the Semont maneuver for the treatment of posterior canal benign paroxysmal positional vertigo. *Journal of Neurology*, *259*, 882-885.

[39] Brandt, T. & Daroff, R. B. (1980). Physical therapy for benign paroxysmal positional vertigo. *Archives of Otolaryngology*, *106*, 484-485.

[40] Kinne, B. L., Crouch, N. A. & Strace, C. L. (2014). Anterior canal benign paroxysmal positional vertigo treatment techniques. *Physical Therapy Reviews*, *19*, 79-85.

[41] Kim, Y. K., Shin, J. E. & Chung, J. W. (2005). The effect of canalith repositioning for anterior semicircular canal canalithiasis. *ORL: Journal for Oto-Rhino-Laryngology and its Related Specialties*, *67*, 56-60.

[42] Yacovino, D. A., Hain, T. C. & Gualtieri, F. (2009). New therapeutic maneuver for anterior canal benign paroxysmal positional vertigo. *Journal of Neurology*, *256*, 1851-1855.

[43] Korres, S., Riga, M., Sandris, V., Danielides, V. & Sismanis, A. (2010). Canalithiasis of the anterior semicircular canal (ASC): Treatment options based on the possible underlying pathogenetic mechanisms. *International Journal of Audiology*, *49*, 606-612.

[44] Casani, A. P., Cerchiai, N., Dallan, I. & Sellari-Franceschini, S. (2011). Anterior canal lithiasis: Diagnosis and treatment. *Otolaryngology: Head and Neck Surgery*, *144*, 412-418.

[45] Kinne, B. L., Strace, C. L. & Crouch, N. A. (2012). The effectiveness of current interventions in the management of lateral canal benign paroxysmal positional vertigo. *Physical Therapy Reviews*, *17*, 292-300.

[46] Asprella-Libonati, G. (2005). Diagnostic and treatment strategy of lateral semicircular canal canalolithiasis. *Acta Otorhinolarngology Italica*, *25*, 277-283.

[47] Casani, A. P., Nacci, A., Dallan, I., Panicucci, E., Gufoni, M. & Sellari-Franceschini, S. (2011). Horizontal semicircular canal benign paroxysmal positional vertigo: Effectiveness of two different methods of treatment. *Audiology and Neurotology*, *16*, 175-184.

[48] Lempert, T. (1994). Horizontal benign positional vertigo. *Neurology*, *44*, 2213-2214.

[49] Sekine, K., Imai, T., Sato, G., Ito, M. & Takeda, N. (2006). Natural history of benign paroxysmal positional vertigo and efficacy of Epley and Lempert maneuvers. *Otolaryngology: Head and Neck Surgery*, *135*, 529-533.

[50] Vannucchi, P., Giannoni, B. & Pagnini, P. (1997). Treatment of horizontal semicircular canal benign paroxysmal positional vertigo. *Journal of Vestibular Research*, *7*, 1-6.

[51] Casani, A. P., Vannucci, G., Fattori, B. & Berrettini, S. (2002). The treatment of horizontal canal positional vertigo: Our experience in 66 cases. *Laryngoscope*, *112*, 172-178.

[52] Oh, S. Y., Kim, J. S., Jeong, S. H., Oh, Y. M., Choi, K. D., Kim, B. K., . Lee, J. J. (2009). Treatment of apogeotropic benign positional vertigo: Comparison of therapeutic head-shaking and modified Semont maneuver. *Journal of Neurology*, *256*, 1330-1336.

In: Eye Movement Disorders
Editor: Sloan L. Mills
ISBN: 978-1-63321-980-9

Chapter 2

Anesthetic Implications of Strabismus Surgery

L. Sean Lawson, CRNA, MSN, ARNP
and Gregory L. Rose, M.D.*
[1]Department of Anesthesiology
University of Kentucky College of Medicine
[2]Associate Professor, Department of Anesthesiology
University of Kentucky College of Medicine Lexington, Kentucky, US

Abstract

The anesthetic implications of eye muscle surgery are varied and numerous. Being a condition that can be seen in all age groups, the anesthetist or anesthesiologist will see pediatric, adult, and geriatric patient populations. Though it may be minimally invasive on an anatomical basis, strabismus surgery can be perhaps surprisingly invasive physiologically because of the oculocardiac reflex, and the clinician needs to be well versed in management and treatment of any cardiac dysrhythmia so that if it occurs, it can be handled instantly and successfully. Since eye muscle surgery is usually done on an outpatient basis, post-operative nausea and vomiting need to be well controlled even

* Email: glrose0@email.uky.edu.

though eye muscle surgery is well known for being very nausea-provoking. Our chapter will focus on these factors in detail.

Introduction

An old maxim among anesthesiologists and nurse anesthetists is "there may be minor surgeries, but no minor anesthetics". This means that even though an operative procedure may be minor, with little to no inherent risk to life or limb, all anesthetics, even local anesthesia, impart some amount of risk that could be life-threatening. We expect anesthesia providers to be vigilant and aware of all potential risks involved with any anesthetic. This is the *standard of care* that those undergoing any medical procedure expect and deserve.

While eye muscle surgery in and of itself is not trivial, the surgical portion carries few risks of loss of life, apart from catastrophic hemorrhage or infection that develops into sepsis. The anesthetic portion however, certainly carries the risk of death, whether the patient is pediatric or adult, healthy or unhealthy. Loss of airway with anoxic brain damage, anaphylaxis, or pulmonary aspiration can occur in eye muscle surgery as easily as it can happen in more invasive surgery.

Apart from the potential risks of all anesthetics, anesthesia for strabismus surgery carries some implications that are, while not totally peculiar to it, are seen more often with it than with other anesthetics.

Strabismus surgery is one of the most common pediatric surgeries, rivalling the numbers for tonsillectomies and myringotomies. It is the most common pediatric ophthalmologic procedure. It is also not an uncommon ophthalmologic procedure in the adult population. This chapter will discuss the anesthetic implications of eye muscle surgery.

Oculocardiac Reflex

As mentioned, strabismus surgery is the most common ophthalmic surgery in the pediatric population. A common adverse event that the anesthetist, anesthesiologist, and ophthalmologist, need to be aware of is the oculocardiac reflex (OCR). These participants in ophthalmic procedures need to be aware of the occurrence of OCR, recognize the clinical manifestations and be proficient in treating it.

OCR was first described in 1908[1]. It occurs with traction of the extraocular muscles. It can also occur with pressure on the globe, conjunctiva, orbital structures and any remaining tissue in the orbit. The reflex may also be elicited from the performance of a retrobulbar block. The reflex may occur under local or general anesthesia and is believed to be augmented by the presence of hypercarbia and hypoxemia. The occurrence of OCR varies, with rates ranging from 16 – 82% [1]. The rates of occurrence vary on the patient population studied and the definition used to determine the reflex. The definition most accepted by most resources defines OCR as a decrease in heart rate greater than 20% from baseline. It is noted to occur at a greater rate in the pediatric population, yet it does occur with frequency in adults.

Although bradycardia is the predominant manifestation, other arrhythmias may occur. Rhythms of note include junctional rhythm, ectopic atrial rhythm, atrioventricular blockade, ventricular bigeminy, multifocal premature ventricular contractions, wandering pacemaker, idioventricular rhythm, ventricular tachycardia, and asystole.

The reflex consists of afferent pathway through the trigeminal nerve and an efferent pathway through the vagus nerve [2]. More specifically the afferent limb travels via the ophthalmic division of the trigeminal nerve. The reflex begins with the long and short ciliary nerves that travel along the ophthalmic division. It continues to the gasserian ganglion and then joins the main sensory pathway of the trigeminal nerve in the floor of the fourth ventricle. Short internuncial pathways connect it to the efferent pathway from the motor nucleus of the vagus nerve. The pathway ends with the depressor fibers of the myocardium.

The risk factors for OCR include hypercapnia, hypoxemia, inadequate general anesthesia, age (the reflex is more pronounced in the pediatric population), surgical stimulus (the strength and duration of traction), and pharmacologic agents [3]. Drugs noted to worsen OCR include beta-blockers, calcium channel blockers and narcotics such as sufentanil and remifentanil. Beta-blockers worsen the reflex by reducing the sympathetic response of the heart and contribute to bradycardia. Calcium channel blockers cause peripheral arterial smooth muscle relaxation resulting in vasodilation and hypotension. Narcotics such as sufentanil and remifentanil will inhibit the sympathetic nervous system thus decreasing vagal tone [3].

Treatment of OCR begins with awareness of the potential occurrence of the reflex [2]. The next step involves notifying the surgeon of the occurrence of the reflex so that temporary cessation of the surgical stimuli may be performed. Most cases of OCR usually resolve with the release of extraocular muscle traction. The next step in treatment is ensuring adequate ventilation (to avoid hypercapnia) and oxygenation are be provided to the patient. Depth of anesthesia should be assessed to determine its effectiveness. Should the reflex continue following these interventions the administration of anticholinergic agents such as atropine or glycopyrrolate may be administered. The dose of atropine found to be adequate is 10 mcg/kg and 0.02 mg/kg for glycopyrrolate. The reflex is fatigable; with the reoccurrence of the reflex, fatigue may occur and it becomes self-limiting [2].

Historically, administration of atropine at induction was much more common in the past with pediatric patients due to the widespread use of the inhalational agent halothane, which commonly caused bradycardia; nevertheless, such use was ineffective in prevention of OCR [1]. Atropine is a myocardial irritant and may lead to more malignant arrhythmias if OCR occurs. Arrhythmias attributed to atropine include ventricular fibrillation, ventricular tachycardia and left bundle branch block.

Anesthetic and Pharmacologic Effects on the Oculocardiac Reflex

Choi et al. noted generalized differences in effect of OCR for a variety of anesthetic techniques. They noted that sevoflurane is associated with a lower occurrence of OCR than propofol. The incidence of OCR was similar with the use of sevoflurane and desflurane. Sufentanil and remifentanil enhanced the severity of bradycardia with their use [4].

A study was performed by Oh et al. comparing the incidence of OCR in the use of sevoflurane versus desflurane. Their study noted that the occurrence of OCR for strabismus surgery with the use of sevoflurane and desflurane were similar. Desflurane is the only agent to increase sympathetic activity. This is believed to occur from stimulation or receptors in or near the airway rather than baroreceptors. This increase in sympathetic activity is more pronounced if desflurane concentration is increased rapidly. The occurrence was 26% versus 28%. They also noted the incidence of OCR was lower in children in the 2-5 age group compared to children in the 6-10 age group [5].

A 2007 study compared single dose ketamine versus propofol for the induction of anesthesia and the occurrence of OCR. Their study noted that the incidence of OCR was lower in those receiving a single bolus of ketamine than with those receiving a propofol induction without an increase in postoperative recovery time. Their study noted that ketamine may reduce the OCR when used with sevoflurane for the maintenance of anesthesia. Ketamine may have sympathomimetic effects and inhibit the parasympathetic reflex of the OCR. Propofol displayed the ability to increase the incidence of bradycardia by a central sympatholytic effect and vagal stimulation [6].

A study by Chung et al. from 2008 looked at the incidence of OCR with use of remifentanil in strabismus surgery. Remifentanil is a potent synthetic opioid with a short duration and stable context sensitive half time. Remifentanil may cause bradycardia by stimulation of the parasympathetic nervous system and also through negative chronotropy. Their study noted that remifentanil displayed an increased incidence of OCR with a more exaggerated decrease in heart rate in comparison to the use of sevoflurane alone [7].

It is important for the clinician to realize that vagal nerve-induced arrhythmias may present from stimulation from any division of the trigeminal nerve. Episodes of cardiac dysrhythmias have been reported during nasal, mandibular, and other maxillofacial procedures [8].

Forced Duction Test

The reader is no doubt familiar with the technique and purpose of the forced duction test (FDC) in eye muscle surgery. It is discussed in other chapters of this book. Among other potential problems with its use in eye muscle surgery, the muscle relaxant succinylcholine (sux) can interfere with the interpretation of the FDC.

Succinylcholine is a *depolarizing* muscle relaxant, which means that on contact with the acetylcholine receptor at the neuromuscular junction, the succinylcholine molecule causes an action potential with contraction of the muscle fiber. This is an example of competitive agonism, whereas the other clinically used muscle relaxants, e.g. rocuronium, vecuronium, atracurium, cis-atracurium, and pancuronium are competitive antagonists, occupying the receptor but causing no action potential. These are classified as *nondepolarizing* muscle relaxants.

The firing of individual muscle fibers is manifested as fasciculations, where the skeletal muscles can be seen fibrillating at random after administration of succinylcholine. These fasciculations usually last less than one minute by gross examination. However, the density of motor endplates in the extraocular muscles is so great that fasciculations after sux can last up to twenty minutes. These can influence the interpretation of the FDC.

The authors have worked with individual ophthalmologists who perform an FDC with each procedure and others who never do. Therefore communication is of value if the surgeon wishes to perform an FDC. Fortunately the use of sux has decreased over the last couple of decades for various reasons; those discussed in the next section, plus the availability of nondepolarizing relaxants with shorter duration of action, and the use of supraglottic airways like the laryngeal mask. It should be rare that sux *must* be used for the vast majority of elective eye procedures.

The Use of Succinylcholine in Strabismus Surgery

For many years the use of succinylcholine (sux) for muscle relaxation to facilitate endotracheal intubation for eye muscle surgery has been rather controversial. One reason given to avoid succinylcholine is related to its possible alteration of the forced duction test. The other reason is out of the concern that patients, especially those in the pediatric population, may have an undiagnosed or latent muscular dystrophy of which strabismus is the only current symptom; administration of succinylcholine to such patients can be potentially life-threatening.

There have been many reports in the literature of infants and children, mostly male, who developed cardiac arrest from sudden catastrophic hyperkalemia and rhabdomyolosis immediately following administration of succinylcholine [9]. In one study that searched the literature, 56% of children survived the arrest, and half of those studied were later found to have an undiagnosed muscle disease [10]. While succinylcholine has long been known to cause hyperkalemia in certain acquired conditions, such as recent third-degree burns, spinal cord injuries, muscle crush injuries as well as genetic muscle diseases such as the muscular dystrophies, these cases of hyperkalemia in infants and children were from *undiagnosed* dystrophies.

Furthermore, a 1993 review of 500 cases of malignant hyperthermia (MH) showed an increased incidence of MH during strabismus surgery compared to other procedures [11]. While there has never been a direct link between the two, some references say that there is an increased risk of malignant hyperthermia in strabismus.

In addition, the Federal Drug Administration (FDA) issued a "black box" warning in 1992 advising about the risk of sudden hyperkalemic cardiac arrest in infants and children following the injection of succinylcholine [12].

Because of these concerns of hyperkalemia in occult dystrophic pediatric patients and the possible increased risk of malignant hyperthermia, as well as the alterations that succinylcholine produces on the forced duction test, most anesthesia providers choose not to use succinylcholine when performing anesthetics for strabismus procedures. There are other muscle relaxants that are nondepolarizing (that do not increase serum potassium levels or trigger MH) that can be used that do not cause the same problems that sux can; their only disadvantage is they all confer muscle relaxation for a time much greater than sux does, (e.g. 5 minutes for sux vs 30 minutes for the quickest nondepolarizing relaxant, rocuronium). Moreover, with the increased use of the laryngeal mask or other supraglottic airways, muscle relaxation is often not needed for airway management.

Anesthetic Techniques

The traditional method of performing an anesthetic for eye muscle surgery was general endotracheal inhalational anesthesia. (Topical anesthesia or blocks have been used in the adult population, but most anesthetists prefer general anesthetic). For the most part, endotracheal intubation necessitates the use of muscle relaxants to facilitate laryngoscopy. This posed a conundrum for clinicians- should the short acting succinylcholine be used and possibly interfere with a forced duction test, or use a nondepolarizing muscle relaxant, none of which can be reversed adequately for at least 30 minutes.

If a procedure was performed relatively quickly, the patient would be unable to breathe on their own until the nondepolarizing relaxant was reversible using anticholinesterase inhibitors, delaying emergence, and causing the room to be delayed as well. Avoiding the use of muscle relaxants for intubation has been common in pediatric practice, but becomes more difficult for adult patients.

The laryngeal mask airway, or supraglottic airway came into general use in the early to mid-1990s. This device quickly gained acceptance among anesthesiologists and anesthetists for airway maintenance for many different procedures, including ophthalmic procedures. By the end of the decade studies using the laryngeal mask specifically for strabismus procedures had been published.

Laryngeal mask airways however, do have certain drawbacks for the clinician. Since it is supraglottic, it is not a secure airway. Aspiration of stomach contents (even in patients who are NPO) is possible with LMAs and this is a disadvantage over cuffed endotracheal tubes. LMAs are more easily dislodged during the procedure, necessitating airway rescue close to an operative field. Administering positive airway pressure of a value over 20-30 cm H_2O can lead to inadvertent insufflation of the stomach, which can increase risk of passive aspiration. It is more difficult to adequately ventilate obese patients with an LMA leading to hypercarbia and hypoxemia due to their restrictive airway pattern. Some surgeons may find the external tube portion of the LMA to impinge on the operating space even if it is under drapes. LMAs with flexible, wire-wound, non-kinking stems are available. But these are not disposable, and are more difficult to place. In our practice, we have found that regular LMAs can be easily bent and taped to not intrude on the operative field without kinking.

Any patient who is at a risk for pulmonary aspiration should be intubated with an endotracheal tube, despite potential difficulties with reversal of muscle relaxation. This includes the morbidly obese, patients with gastroparesis, symptomatic gastroesophageal reflux disease, and recently postpartum patients. Patients with full stomachs should be postponed until they meet NPO status, the time of which is dependent on the type of food eaten.

While total intravenous anesthesia (TIVA) with propofol lessens the overall incidence of post-operative nausea and vomiting (PONV), inhalational anesthesia is still used regularly for eye muscle procedures. The use of narcotics, while necessary for postoperative comfort, is minimized with the addition of non-narcotic analgesics such as acetaminophen (oral, rectal, or intravenous administration), and ketorolac. Perioperative pain management is discussed in the next section.

Post-Operative Nausea and Vomiting (PONV)

Ocular procedures, and specifically strabismus procedures, have long been well known causes of postoperative nausea and vomiting (PONV), both in the pediatric and adult populations. In pediatric literature, the problem is referred to usually as postoperative vomiting (POV) since it may be hard to elicit the symptom of nausea from infants and small children. Literally dozens of papers have been written about this subject, and the findings can be confusing, since some were written decades ago using drugs that are no longer available, and not using modern antiemetics.

The rate of PONV or POV following strabismus surgery has been quoted in multiple studies as being anywhere from 30 to 70%, or even higher if no antiemetic therapy is given. Instead of an actual number, we will say that POV/PONV after eye muscle surgery is the norm, and is greatly dependent on several things which are discussed later in this section. Apart from the suffering caused by it, PONV increases the cost of outpatient medical care by prolonging time in the recovery room before discharge, and it is the leading cause of unforeseen hospital admissions after strabismus procedures [3, 13].

Various theories exist for why eye muscle procedures cause PONV independent of the anesthetic technique. Manipulation of the eye muscles and subsequent input to the vestibular system is postulated. Postoperative visual changes leading to nausea is another possibility. Some speak of the oculo-emetic reflex, analogous to the oculo-cardiac reflex (OCR), which induces PONV using the trigeminal nerve as the afferent limb to nausea centers in the brain [14]. Indeed, some studies show a relationship to PONV postoperatively to OCR occurring intraoperatively [15].

PONV is more common for pediatric patients than adult patients following eye muscle surgery. Children over the age of three are at greater risk of POV than younger children, as well as children who have a history of POV and/or motion sickness. Length of procedure (longer than 30 minutes) has been shown to increase the incidence of PONV [16]. In adults, being female and being a nonsmoker are risk factors [17]. The type of anesthetics used is also a factor. Some anesthetics are more emetogenic than others, even in the case of strabismus surgery which is highly nausea provoking in its own right. Nitrous oxide [17], opiates, etomidate, and possibly muscle relaxant reversal agents [18] (anticholinesterase inhibitors, e.g. neostigmine) are known to produce PONV.

Multiple studies have shown that the intravenous anesthetic propofol is superior to inhalational agents and nitrous oxide in the prevention or diminishment of PONV [3]. However, inhalational agents are much simpler to use than propofol infusions, especially in a busy ambulatory center. In adults, the use of local anesthetic blocks to avoid a general anesthetic decreases

PONV. Opiate analgesics can cause PONV, and therefore their use should be limited.

Treatment of PONV can be thought of in two ways; *prevention* of PONV, vs. *treatment of existing* PONV. Prophylactic use of antiemetics is definitely better than waiting until an episode of PONV occurs postoperatively [19]. A study in 2002 in the British Journal of Anaesthesia showed prophylactic use of ondansetron 0.1 mg/kg during the anesthetic can reduce POV in children better than waiting until symptoms of nausea and vomiting occur in the recovery room, as well as reducing time spent in recovery before discharge [20]. Another study of the use of prophylactic ondansetron revealed that 0.07 mg/kg was as effective as 0.15 mg/kg [21].

Another example of PONV prophylaxis is proper hydration. Intravenous "superhydration" with 30 ml/kg of crystalloid decreased PONV in children undergoing strabismus repair compared to a group that received only 10 ml/kg of intravenous crystalloid [22].

Dexamethasone is also an effective antiemetic when given prophylactically. Various doses have been studied, from 0.15 mg/kg to 0.5 mg/kg, and all were effective; 0.25 mg/kg was shown to be as effective as 0.5 mg/kg [23]. Fears of delayed wound healing or postoperative hyperglycemia have not come to pass. Any diabetic should have a postoperative glucose level checked regardless [24]. Some studies have actually presented data that dexamethasone *shortened* wound healing time [25].

Currently, it is believed that combination prophylactic therapy is superior to any single medication used prophylactically, specifically the combination of ondansetron and dexamethasone [3]. Dexamethasone is given on induction of general anesthesia, and ondansetron given at the end of the anesthetic. In general, this applies to cases that are longer than the usual strabismus operation so timing is not as critical as in procedures that last hours.

Metoclopramide is a gastrokinetic drug that has been used a great deal in the past for its antiemetic effects. Its use is much rarer now as an antiemetic because of the superiority of dexamethasone and ondansetron. Each is superior separately to metoclopramide, and are far superior when given in combination [11]. Metoclopramide also has potential adverse side effects not seen in other commonly used antiemetics, such as akathisia, with motor restlessness and feelings of impending doom. There are many case reports of patients who refuse to proceed with surgery after administration of metoclopramide preoperatively [26].

Another antiemetic that was once frequently used is droperidol. Until the United States Food and Drug Administration (FDA) issued a black box warning for it in 2001, droperidol was perhaps the most frequently used perioperative antiemetic, either alone or in combination with another antiemetic [27]. The FDA warning concerned the possibility of Q-T elongation on electrocardiogram, and possible torsade de pointes. However, this risk of dysrhythmias was for dosages in excess of 5 mg, and the usual adult dose of droperidol for antiemesis is 0.625 mg [28]. But because of the black box warning, many institutions stopped stocking the drug, and its use is minimal currently in the United States, compared to what it once was.

Most clinicians attempt to limit the use of narcotics as analgesics. Topical anesthetic drops have not shown to be effective in children for adequate analgesia. A 2011 study showed that IV paracetamol is an effective analgesic and also lowers the incidence of PONV [29]. Dexmetatomidine, a relatively new sedative-hypnotic, was shown in a recent study to decrease PONV [30]. Ketorolac is also useful as an analgesic adjunct in order to lessen the use of opiates, and has been shown not to increase postoperative bleeding, except in the case of tonsillectomies.

References

[1] Barash PG, Cullen BF, Stoelting RK, Cahalan MK, Stock MC, Ortega R, Clinical Anesthesia, 7th edition, Philadelphia: Lippincott Williams and Wilkins, 2013;1379-80.

[2] Butterworth JF, Mackey DC, Wasnick JD, Morgan and Mikhail's Clinical Anesthesiology, 5th edition, McGraw – Hill, 2013; 761-2.

[3] Rodgers A, Cox RG. Anesthetic management for pediatric strabismus surgery: Continuing professional development. *Can J. Anaesth.* 2010;57:602-17.

[4] Choi SR, Park SW, Lee JH, Lee SC, Chung CJ. Effect of different anesthetic agents on oculocardiac reflex in pediatric strabismus surgery. *J. Anesth.* 2009;23:489-93.

[5] Oh AY, Yun MJ, Kim HJ, Kim HS. Comparison of desflurane with sevoflurane for the incidence of oculocardiac reflex in children undergoing strabismus surgery. *Br. J. Anaesth.* 2007;99:262-5.

[6] Choi SH, Lee SJ, Kim SH, Kim JH, Kwon HH, Shin YS, Lee KY. Single bolus of intravenous ketamine for anesthetic induction decreases oculocardiac reflex in children undergoing strabismus surgery. *Acta Anaesthesiol. Scand.* 2007;51:759-62.

[7] Chung CJ, Lee JM, Choi SR, Lee SC, Lee JH. Effect of remifentanil on oculocardiac reflex in paediatric strabismus surgery. *Acta Anaesthesiol. Scand.* 2008;52:1273-7.

[8] Locke MM, Spiekermann BF, Rich GF. Trigeminovagal reflex during repair of a nasal fracture under general anesthesia. *Anesth. Analg.* 1999;88:1183-4.

[9] Rosenberg H, Gronert GA. Intractable cardiac arrest in children given succinylcholine. *Anesthesiology*. 1992;77:1054.

[10] Larach MG, Rosenberg H, Gronert GA, Allen GC. Hyperkalemic cardiac arrest during anesthesia in infants and children with occult myopathies. *Clin. Pediatr* (Phila). 1997;36:9-16.

[11] Strazis KP, Fox AW. Malignant hyperthermia: a review of published cases. *Anesth. Analg*. 1993;77:297-304.

[12] Succinylcholine Black Box Warning. http://www.accessdata.fda.gov/drugsatfda_docs/label/2010/008845s065lbl.pdf. Last Accessed 6-2-14

[13] Elder M, Steven D, Beasley S, Wium D. Unplanned overnight hospital admission after strabismus surgery. *N. Z. Med. J.* 2007;120:U2681.

[14] Gan TJ. Postoperative nausea and vomiting--can it be eliminated? *JAMA*. 2002;287:1233-6.

[15] Allen LE, Sudesh S, Sandramouli S, Cooper G, McFarlane D, Willshaw HE. The association between the oculocardiac reflex and post-operative vomiting in children undergoing strabismus surgery. *Eye* (Lond). 1998;12 (Pt 2):193-6.

[16] Gan TJ. Risk factors for postoperative nausea and vomiting. *Anesth. Analg.* 2006;102:1884-98.

[17] Hartung J. Twenty-four of twenty-seven studies show a greater incidence of emesis associated with nitrous oxide than with alternative anesthetics. *Anesth. Analg*. 1996;83:114-6.

[18] Cheng CR, Sessler DI, Apfel CC. Does neostigmine administration produce a clinically important increase in postoperative nausea and vomiting? *Anesth. Analg*. 2005;101:1349-55.

[19] Gan TJ, Meyer TA, Apfel CC, Chung F, Davis PJ, Habib AS, Hooper VD, Kovac AL, Kranke P, Myles P, Philip BK, Samsa G, Sessler DI, Temo J, Tramèr MR, Vander Kolk C, Watcha M; Society for Ambulatory Anesthesia. Society for Ambulatory Anesthesia guidelines for the management of postoperative nausea and vomiting. *Anesth. Analg.* 2007;105:1615-28.

[20] Sennaraj B, Shende D, Sadhasivam S, Ilavajady S, Jagan D. Management of post-strabismus nausea and vomiting in children using

ondansetron: a value-based comparison of outcomes. *Br. J. Anaesth.* 2002;89:473-8.

[21] Sadhasivam S, Shende D, Madan R. Prophylactic ondansetron in prevention of postoperative nausea and vomiting following pediatric strabismus surgery: a dose-response study. *Anesthesiology.* 2000;92:1035-42.

[22] Goodarzi M, Matar MM, Shafa M, Townsend JE, Gonzalez I. A prospective randomized blinded study of the effect of intravenous fluid therapy on postoperative nausea and vomiting in children undergoing strabismus surgery. *Paediatr Anaesth.* 2006;16:49-53.

[23] Madan R, Bhatia A, Chakithandy S, Subramaniam R, Rammohan G, Deshpande S, Singh M, Kaul HL. Prophylactic dexamethasone for postoperative nausea and vomiting in pediatric strabismus surgery: a dose ranging and safety evaluation study. *Anesth. Analg.* 2005;100:1622-6.

[24] Holte K, Kehlet H. Perioperative single-dose glucocorticoid administration: pathophysiologic effects and clinical implications. *J. Am. Coll Surg.* 2002;195:694-712.

[25] Salerno A, Hermann R. Efficacy and safety of steroid use for postoperative pain relief. Update and review of the medical literature. *J . Bone Joint Surg. Am.* 2006;88:1361-72.

[26] LaGorio J, Thompson VA, Sternberg D, Dorje P. Akathisia and anesthesia: refusal of surgery after the administration of metoclopramide. *Anesth. Analg.* 1998;87:224-7.

[27] Shende D, Bharti N, Kathirvel S, Madan R. Combination of droperidol and ondansetron reduces PONV after pediatric strabismus surgery more than single drug therapy. *Acta Anaesthesiol. Scand.* 2001;45:756-60.

[28] Kao LW, Kirk MA, Evers SJ, Rosenfeld SH. Droperidol, QT prolongation, and sudden death: what is the evidence? *Ann. Emerg. Med.* 2003;41:546-58.

[29] Cok OY, Eker HE, Pelit A, Canturk S, Akin S, Aribogan A, Arslan G. The effect of paracetamol on postoperative nausea and vomiting during the first 24 h after strabismus surgery: a prospective, randomised, double-blind study. *Eur. J. Anaesthesiol.* 2011;28:836-41.

[30] Chen JY, Jia JE, Liu TJ, Qin MJ, Li WX. Comparison of the effects of dexmedetomidine, ketamine, and placebo on emergence agitation after strabismus surgery in children. *Can. J. Anaesth.* 2013;60:385-92.

In: Eye Movement Disorders
Editor: Sloan L. Mills

ISBN: 978-1-63321-980-9

Chapter 3

Central Positional Dizziness

João Lemos, MD[1*] and Eric Eggenberger, DO, MSEpi[2]

[1]Department of Neurology, Coimbra University Hospital Center, Praceta Mota Pinto, Coimbra, Portugal

[2]Department of Neurology & Ophthalmology, Michigan State University, Clinical Center, East Lansing, MI, US

Abstract

While positional dizziness is most commonly related to peripheral vestibular disease, it may rarely be caused by a pontomedullary or vestibulocerebellar lesion. Three main clinical forms have been described: central positional nystagmus (CPN), central paroxysmal positional vertigo (CPPV), and rotational vertebral artery syndrome (RVAS). The first type consists of prolonged positional nystagmus with no or only slight vertigo (e.g. pure downbeat nystagmus in head-hanging position) and seems to be precipitated by a strategic lesion in the cerebellar nodulus and uvula. The second type comprises short-lasting nystagmus combined with vertigo and is provoked by lesions dorsolateral to the fourth ventricle, in the cerebellar vermis or superior cerebellar peduncle. The mechanism by which such lesions cause positional nystagmus seems to involve a vestibular tone imbalance promoted by

* Correspondence to João Lemos, MD, Department of Neurology, Coimbra University Hospital Center, Praceta Mota Pinto, 3000-075 Coimbra, Portugal; Tel: +351 964 319 380; Fax: +351 239 822 637; Email: merrin72@hotmail.com.

disruption of the central otolithic connections between the vestibular nuclei and vestibular cerebellum. Typical causes for CPN and CPPV include haemorrhage, tumour, demyelination, infarction, Chiari malformation and cerebellar degeneration. Vestibular migraine and drug intoxication should also be considered, especially when imaging is normal. The main differential diagnosis of CPPV is benign paroxysmal positional vertigo (BPPV), and given the potentially serious prognosis of infratentorial lesions, this is a critical distinction. Positional nystagmus beating in a plane inconsistent with head and semicircular canal stimulation or purely vertical or torsional should raise suspicion of a central lesion; other features that favor a central origin include absent latency, fatigability and habituation on repetitive stimulation, positional or positioning nystagmus without vertigo, positioning-induced vomiting without nystagmus, and additional cerebellar and oculomotor signs. A third type of central positional dizziness is caused by dynamic compression of one vertebral artery as a result of head rotation (RVAS) promoting transient ischemia of the cerebellum and/or labyrinth, with resultant nystagmus and vertigo. Untreated RVAS may lead to posterior circulation stroke.

Keywords: Vertigo, central positional nystagmus, central paroxysmal positional/positioning vertigo, rotational vertebral artery syndrome

Introduction

Nystagmus and/or vertigo can be specifically triggered by certain head positions or changes in head position. Most cases are due to peripheral vestibular lesions; however, occasionally, a central nervous system (CNS) lesion may be the culprit. Central positional dizziness (CPD) refers to a variety of CNS vestibular syndromes that manifest as positional/positioning nystagmus and/or vertigo, and are caused by posterior fossa lesions that disrupt otolithic inputs from the inner ear to cerebellum. In one series of 100 patients with positional vertigo and/or nystagmus, 12% had central positional dizziness [1]. Otolithic organs lying in the inner ear (the utricule and saccule) are activated in response to linear accelerations and/or changes in head positions in space, sending information to the cerebellum directly or via the vestibular nuclei [2]. Once the head is brought into an off-vertical position, a change in otolithic input is assumed to precipitate pathological CPD. Moreover, based on the fact that this input modulates different subsystems concerning eye movement control (e.g., integrator system, burst generator system), it has been hypothesized that a mismatch between the otolithic information arriving to these different subsystems may cause CPD [3]. Although no current theory can uniformly explain the pathophysiology of CPD, lesions involving the otolithic circuits between the cerebellum and vestibular nuclei are believed to cause central positional nystagmus and/or vertigo by releasing the vestibular nuclei from cerebellar inhibition [4]. Additionally, transient ischemia of the peripheral labyrinth may account for rare cases in which head rotation with subsequent compression of one vertebral artery is believed to induce nystagmus and vertigo [5].

Three main types of CPD can be delineated, according to their clinical features [6, 7]:

1. Central positional nystagmus (CPN)
2. Central paroxysmal positional/positioning vertigo (CPPV)
3. Rotational vertebral artery syndrome (RVAS)

The first two forms mainly differ in terms of their temporal features and the presence of associated perceptual and/or autonomic symptoms: CPN presents with nystagmus that usually persists as long as the precipitant head position is maintained, with little or no vertigo [8]; CPPV usually manifests with short-lasting positional or positioning nystagmus, vertigo and vomiting, of which the latter may dominate the clinical picture [9]. It should be noted however that a clear distinction between these two clinical subtypes is not always possible as patients with persistent positional nystagmus associated with intense vertigo or vomiting, and short-lasting positional nystagmus with no vertigo or vomiting have been reported [10-12]. Rarely, both types co-exist in the same patient, either simultaneously or in a sequential fashion [13, 14]. While CPN is usually easy to differentiate from its peripheral counterpart, benign paroxysmal positioning vertigo (BPPV), CPPV may simulate BPPV, especially if additional oculomotor signs such as saccadic pursuit and gaze-evoked nystagmus are lacking [6]. Finally, CPN has to be distinguished from augmentation of existing spontaneous nystagmus which has been transiently enhanced by a change in head position (e.g., downbeat nystagmus which increases in supine or head-hanging position); these two conditions probably imply different underlying pathophysiology and lesion location [15-18]. Regarding the third type of central positional dizziness, rotational vertebral artery syndrome, the pathophysiology differs from that of CPN and CPPV. While in the latter two, inflammatory, ischemic, compressive or degenerative lesions directly affect the central vestibular system, in RVAS, dynamic compression of one vertebral artery is believed to cause transient ischemia of the central and/or peripheral vestibular system [7].

Central Positional Nystagmus

Persistent nystagmus without vertigo has a central origin until proven otherwise (central positional nystagmus) [19, 20]. Overall, CPN is rare, constituting 1% of patients observed in a neuro-otology clinic [21]. Nevertheless, if one only considers a subpopulation of patients with posterior fossa tumors, CPN prevalence radically increases up to 90% of patients [19]. It can usually be elicited in the supine position with the head centered, rotated right or left or with neck extension off the edge, and in the standing or seated position with the neck flexed or extended. Importantly, in about 40% of cases CPN can only be demonstrated in the head-hanging position [21]. The directional patterns of nystagmus in CPN include oblique, torsional, vertical or horizontal geotropic/apogeotropic with head rotations while supine, and pure downbeat in the head-hanging position, the latter two patterns being the most frequent (Figure 1) [8, 15, 22].

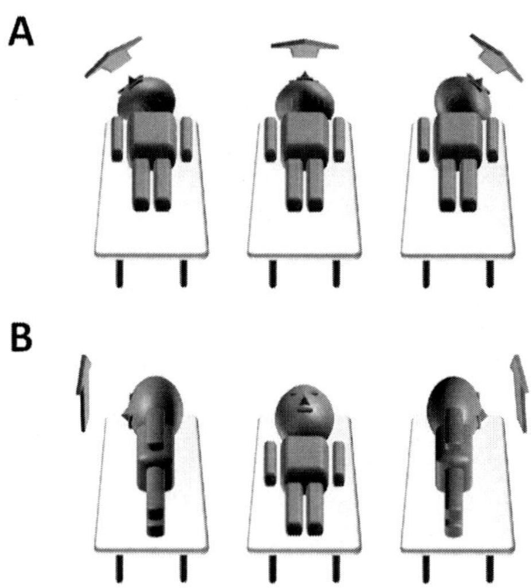

Figure 1. Central positional nystagmus. A. Downbeat nystagmus in right, left and centered head-hanging position; B. Horizontal ageotropic nystagmus in left and right head turn while in supine position [8, 15]. The arrow's direction represents fast phase direction of nystagmus.

Contrary to BPPV, nystagmus in CPN usually shows no latency after the precipitating maneuver and does not fatigue after repeated positional testing [8]. The slow velocity phase of the nystagmus is usually constant in opposition to the crescendo-decrescendo pattern seen in BPPV due to canalithiasis [23]. Since many of the clinical studies reporting the occurrence of CPN were performed before more sophisticated imaging techniques became available, the precise location of the lesion responsible for CPN is still unknown [15]. It has been hypothesized that caudal brainstem and cerebellar lesions may cause CPN [22].

This view has been corroborated by animal experimental data evidencing positional supine downbeat nystagmus after nodulus and uvula ablation in cats, possibly reflecting a release of vestibular nuclei from cerebellar inhibition [24, 25].

Interestingly, bilateral labyrinthectomy abolished positional nystagmus in these experiments [24]. Additionally, recent case reports describing patients with focal strategic cerebellar nodular lesions have shed some light on the pathophysiology of CPN [8, 26]. A lesion affecting this structure possibly impairs transduction of the otolithic signal, this way promoting defective modulation of semicircular canal-ocular reflexes, of which the nodulus is known to inhibit, and subsequent failure of the eyes to readjust their position within the orbit during changes in head position [3, 27]. Etiologies accounting for CPN encompass cerebellar tumors and metastasis, infarction, multiple sclerosis, cranio-cervical malformation, cerebellar degeneration including multiple system atrophy and spinocerebellar ataxia type 6, and vestibular migraine [8, 10, 15, 23, 28-32]. Apart from pathological states, it is noteworthy that up to 70% of asymptomatic healthy individuals may exhibit positional low velocity nystagmus in the dark [33]. Indeed, this type of nystagmus may also reverse its direction in accord with changes in head position and may show horizontal, vertical, torsional or oblique orientation, similarly to CPN [33, 34].

Characteristically, thys this physiological nystagmus abates in light and accordingly should not be present under Frenzel lenses [35]. This normal phenomenon may reflect the physiological “noise” originated from a hypothetical internal network that helps to estimate gravity and linear acceleration in different head orientations in space [36]. In CPN, this network can become deranged, leading to overt positional nystagmus.

Central Paroxysmal Positional/Positioning Vertigo

Short-lasting positional vertigo and/or vomiting and accompanying nystagmus are commonly caused by peripheral semicircular canal disease; however, if vertigo and/or vomiting are prominent and severe and/or atypical direction, latency or duration of nystagmus is noted, an underlying cerebellar disorder may be found in up to 30% of the cases [20]. The latter situation is termed central paroxysmal positional/positioning vertigo; because it may clinically mimic BPPV, CPPV is also called pseudo-BPPV [37]. Importantly, CPPV can be the first and sole presenting feature of central nervous system disease [4].

Nevertheless, accompanying symptoms and signs are frequently encountered and these include gait and posture difficulties, falls, slurred speech, orthostatic intolerance, urinary dysfunction, cerebellar ocular motor abnormalities, and autonomic, pyramidal and extrapyramidal system findings [17]. As in CPN, CPPV can be elicited by bringing the head into an off-vertical, lateral or head-hanging position, either by performing a rapid head movement in which the movement itself can promote *positioning* nystagmus, or by slowly moving the head into a new position which causes *positional* nystagmus.

Although in particular patients the distinction between positioning and positional nystagmus can be challenging based on bedside assessment, this classification is extremely important from an etiological perspective, since it allows the separation between central velocity storage or peripheral semicircular canal disorders (positioning) and central otolithic network or peripheral cupular disorders (positional) [38]. Nystagmus in CPPV can be purely torsional, horizontal geotropic and ageotropic, or vertical, mainly downbeat (Figure 2) [4, 37, 39-42].

Rarely, geotropic horizontal nystagmus can reverse its direction while the head is maintained in the lateral position, transforming into an apogeotropic form, supine upbeat nystagmus can reverse to downbeat nystagmus, or can periodically alternate between each other [1, 10, 43]. In CPPV, strategic focal lesions have been found in the dorsolateral wall of the fourth ventricle, dorsal vermis, nodulus and uvula, superior cerebellar peduncle and prepositus hypoglossi nucleus (Figure 3) [4, 6, 10, 39, 41, 42, 44, 45].

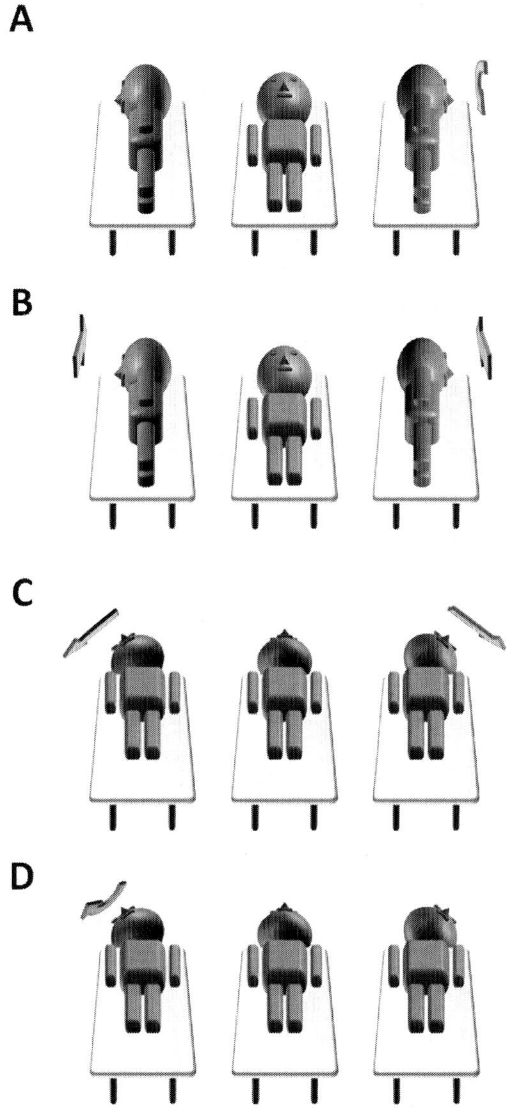

Figure 2. Central paroxysmal positional/positioning vertigo. A. Left torsional nystagmus in left head turn, while in supine position; B. Upbeat nystagmus in right and left head turn, while in supine position; C. Horizontal geotropic nystagmus in right and left head-hanging position; D. Right torsional nystagmus in right head-hanging position [4, 42]. The arrow's direction represents fast phase direction of nystagmus. The direction of torsional nystagmus corresponds to the fast movement direction of the superior pole of the eyes, being considered from the patient's perspective.

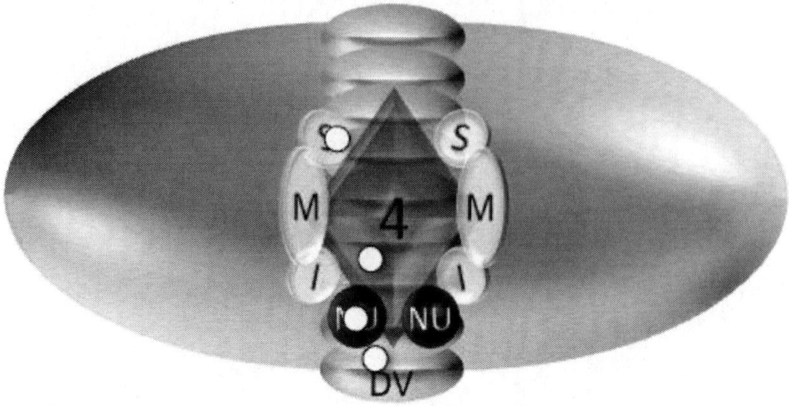

Figure 3. Schematic drawing of cerebellum highlighting strategic lesions (white dots) causing central positional nystagmus and central paroxysmal positional/positioning vertigo. S, superior cerebellar peduncle; M, middle cerebellar peduncle; I, inferior cerebellar peduncle; 4, fourth ventricle; NU, nodulus and uvula; DV, dorsal vermis.

Computed tomography (CT) scan is associated with a low sensitivity for posterior fossa infarction, and accordingly the clinician should be aware that a causative lesion often eludes detection by head CT in a patient with CPPV [4]. Rarely, the brain magnetic resonance imaging (MRI) may fail to demonstrate the causative lesion [42]; however, this is not uncommon if imaging is done acutely [46]. In a few cases, only 2-deoxy-2-[F18]fluoro-D-glucose-positron emission tomography (FDG-PET) provides evidence of cerebellar nodular dysfunction [47]. The nodulus inhibits velocity storage mechanisms during rapid head tilts. The mechanism of CPPV, at least in the positioning forms, may be related to impaired vestibulocerebellar inhibition of the brainstem velocity storage or its inputs from the vestibulo-ocular reflex VOR signals [38, 48]. An instability of the velocity storage system may explain the rare CPPV type showing spontaneous reversion in the direction of positional nystagmus possibly trying to nullify abnormally long duration nystagmus [43]. Not mutually exclusive, a lesion in the inner portion of the superior cerebellar peduncle may induce disruption of the central otolithic connections between cerebellum and the vestibular nuclei [39, 41, 44]. All these mechanisms will ultimately promote disinhibition of archicerebello-vestibular efferents not only to the ocular motor structures concerning the vestibulo-ocular reflex (nystagmus and vertigo) but also to the area postrema area and lateral reticular formation (vomiting) [40]. There are numerous causes of CPPV including posterior fossa tumors, brainstem infarction and hemorrhage, multiple sclerosis, evstibular vestibular migraine and less commonly, paraneoplastic, intoxication (e.g., amiodarone, pregabalin), multiple system atrophy, spinocerebellar ataxia type 6, hydrocephalus, cranio-cervical malformation, and infratentorial arachnoid cyst [4, 17, 29, 37, 40, 45, 47, 49-51]. Vestibular migraine diagnosis should be considered in CPPV patients evidencing repeated positional attacks of nausea and vertigo and low velocity sustained nystagmus without latency, in whom serial imaging studies are consistently normal and repositioning maneuvers do not seem to be effective [29]. Even in the inter-ictal period, asymptomatic positional nystagmus may be found in these patients, and may provide an additional clue to vestibular migraine [14]. The diagnosis of vestibular migraine can be challenging when associated migrainous symptoms such as headache and photophobia are lacking during the attack, as they often are [14]. In the presence of normal brain magnetic resonance imaging (MRI), intoxication and a paraneoplastic syndrome should also be considered [40, 47]. Cranio-cervical malformation, while representing a frequent cause for spontaneous downbeat nystagmus, rarely promotes CPPV [16, 17, 50]. The reason for this discrepancy probably lies in the fact that in CCM there is preferential impairment of cerebellar flocculus/paraflocculus, an area believed to be involved in the generation of spontaneous downbeat nystagmus, while the nodulus and uvula seem to be spared, thus explaining the rare occurrence of positional downbeat nystagmus [17].

Concerning treatment, the only evidence comes from anedoctal reports. Considerable benefit was shown in a recent case report with the use of 4-amynopiridine (4-AP), which abolished recurrent positional downbeat nystagmus (DBN) in a patient with a posterior vermian lesion [52]. The authors hypothesized that this drug induced reactivation of nodulus and (para-) flocculus. Indeed, treatment with 4-AP attenuated abnormally increased regional cerebral glucose metabolism (rCGM) in these areas when using a [18F]-fluorodeoxyglucose-(FDG)-PET protocol. In another patient, a small positive effect of 3,4-aminopyridine (3,4-AP) on positioning DBN was noted [48]. In both cases, 3,4-AP possibly restored the deficient uvulo-nodular inhibition. In another subset of patients evidencing a genetic form of degenerative ataxia, the use of acetazolamide lessened the episodes of positional vertigo with central positional nystagmus and episodic ataxia [51]. Acetazolamide effect was probably mediated through stabilization of the transient dysfunction of calcium channels in the cerebellum. Regarding anecdotal cases of paraneoplastic CPPV, tumor removal, chemotherapy and radiotherapy have shown a modest or no effect on CPPV [53, 54].

Due to the substantial clinical overlap between CPPV and BVVPBPPV, a few points deserve further discussion:

- Using features such as latency, duration and fatigability of nystagmus to separate CPPV from BPPV may prove to be ineffective in individual cases, because all these parameters can vary substantially among CPPV patients. Nevertheless, a prolonged duration of nystagmus and absence of latency and fatigability should raise the suspicion for CNS disease [4, 37, 45, 55].
- On the contrary, the direction of nystagmus can be crucial for making a correct diagnosis: pure vertical or torsional nystagmus, occurring regardless of specific head position or provocative maneuvers indicates a central lesion until proven otherwise. This premise does not follow without warning, since BPPV of the anterior semicircular canal due to canalolithiasis can present with strictly vertical nystagmus lacking the characteristic torsional component [17, 42].
- The direction of nystagmus not obeying the direction of the canal being stimulated by the provocative maneuver (i.e., horizontal for the horizontal canal and vertical-torsional for the vertical canals (Figure 4)) is another indicator of CNS dysfunction (e.g., upbeat nystagmus when the head is in a supine position and rotated to the left) [42].
- Certain presentations are known to be associated with CNS disease, including the presence of downbeat nystagmus only in the head-hanging position, intense vomiting with slight or no nystagmus and the presence of headache aggravated by the Valsalva maneuver. These features should be considered atypical for BPPV and prompt further studies [4, 9, 40, 55].
- CPPV may simulate horizontal canal BPPV; however, "red flags" including positional nystagmus only triggered to one side, associated neurologic symptoms or signs, and unchanged (from ageotropic to geotropic) nystagmus after repositioning maneuvers should raise suspicion for a central disorder. In the appropriate context, alternativee diagnosis should be ruled out, including endolymphatic hydrops, vestibular schwannoma, unilateral or bilateral vestibulopathy, alcohol-related positional nystagmus, and autoimmune inner ear disease [8, 56-59].
- CPPV can also mimic anterior canal BPPV. In this scenario, the co-existence of spontaneous nystagmus and the absence of latency or fatigability of nystagmus demands further investigation in search of a

central etiology [17, 23]. The presence or absence of a torsional component in positional downbeat nystagmus does not reliably differentiate CPPB from BPPV [17].

- Sustained nystagmus with positional testing in a young to middle-aged adult patient presenting with vertigo, nausea and headache and normal MRI should raise the possibility of vestibular migraine [29].

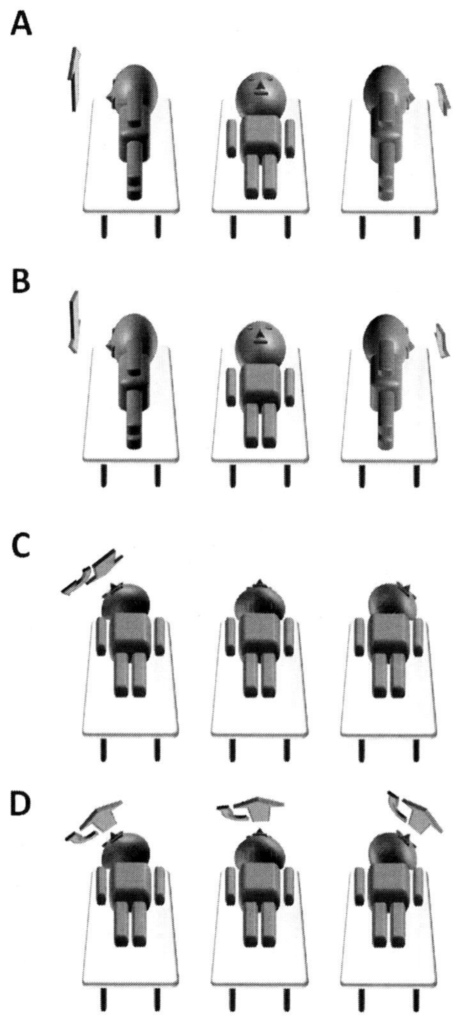

Figure 4. Benign paroxysmal positional/positioning vertigo. A. Horizontal ageotropic nystagmus in right and left head turn, while in supine position: BPPV due to cupulolithiasis of the left horizontal semicircular canal; (Continued on next page)

B. Horizontal geotropic nystagmus in right and left head turn, while in supine position: BPPV due to canalolithiasis of the right horizontal semicircular canal; C. Upbeat and right torsional nystagmus in the right head-hanging position: BPPV due to canalolithiasis of the right posterior semicircular canal; D. Downbeat and right torsional nystagmus in the right, centered and left head-hanging position: BPPV due to canalolithiasis of the right anterior semicircular canal. Note: anterior semicircular canal BPPV can also be triggered in the centered and contralateral head-hanging position due to the particular anatomical orientation of the ampullary segment of the anterior canal, allowing parallel and *orthogonal* rotations to the plane of the canal to provoke anterior semicircular VPPB BPPV [17, 60]. The arrow's direction represents fast phase direction of nystagmus. The direction of torsional nystagmus corresponds to the fast movement direction of the superior pole of the eyes, being considered from the patient's perspective. Smaller arrows represent less intense nystagmus.

Rotational Vertebral Artery Syndrome

Recurrent episodes of paroxysmal vertigo, nystagmus and ataxia induced exclusively by horizontal head rotation constitute a unique and rare form of CPD. Rotational vertebral artery syndrome is supposedly caused by kinking and stretching of one vertebral artery (VA) in the presence of concomitant stenosis or anomaly of the other, leading to haemodynamic ischemia in the vertebrobasilar territory [7]. When the head is rotated to one side, the contralateral VA is usually compressed against an osteophyte, fibrous band, soft tissue, facet joint, or bony prominence, usually at C1-C2 level, causing decrease or cessation of blood flow [61]. Probably, the more anatomic obstacles are present, the less the degree of head turning necessary to cause symptoms [62]. Besides vertigo and/or nystagmus, patients may also evidence tinnitus, presyncope, syncope, headache, blurred vision, sensorimotor disturbance and/or amaurosis fugax during the episodes [5, 61, 63-66]. Interestingly, only a minority of patients report nausea or vomiting [66]. Although RVAS is a rare condition, it may be an ominous sign of impending VA occlusion [67]. Therefore, early diagnosis and proper management are of outmost importance. The most common form of nystagmus in RVAS is mixed downbeat and horizontal, with or without a torsional component, but pure upbeat and downbeat nystagmus have also been described (Figure 5) [63-69].

Nystagmus may reverse or habituate [64, 66]. Initially there is usually a latent period of several seconds [63, 65-69]. The duration of nystagmus is variable, although characteristically patients do not tolerate vertigo beyond 5 to 10 seconds after the head rotation and turn their heads back to a neutral position to alleviate symptoms [5, 63-69].

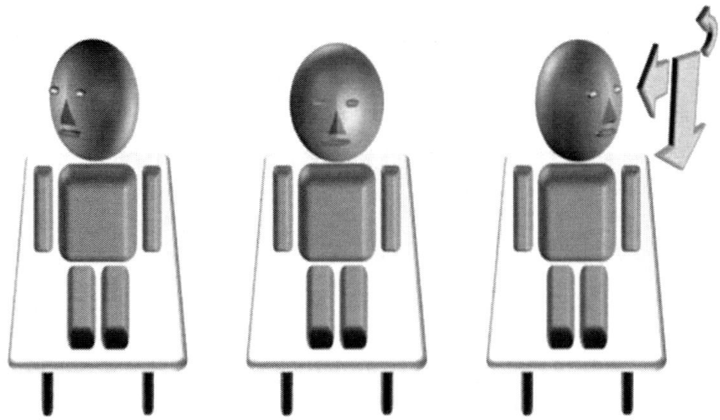

Figure 5. Rotational vertebral artery syndrome. Downbeat and right horizontal and torsional nystagmus in left head turn, while in the seated position, due to dynamic compression of the right vertebral artery [66]. The arrow's direction represents fast phase direction of nystagmus. The direction of torsional nystagmus corresponds to the fast movement direction of the superior pole of the eyes, being considered from the patient's perspective.

Head rotation to one side is the provocative maneuver in the majority of cases, and elicitation of nystagmus with bilateral head rotation or tilt to one side is exceedingly rare [66]. Evaluation using dynamic angiography (during progressive head rotation to the symptomatic side) is the standard method of diagnosis, disclosing stenosis or complete occlusion of one vertebral artery, usually at C2 level [7, 63, 68, 69]. Non-invasive techniques such as CT angiography and transcranial Doppler can be used as an initial screening tool to select patients for a dynamic angiogram and may eventually replace conventional angiography in selected cases where it is contraindicated [67, 70].

Brain MRI and cerebral angiography, CT or MR angiography with the head in the neutral position are usually normal except for the presence of hypoplasia, stenosis, occlusion or anomalous origin of the other vertebral artery [63]. Part of the mechanism causing RVAS is still a matter of debate. While some authors favor transient asymmetric ischemia of the peripheral labyrinth, others suggest a cerebellar and/or brainstem ischemic process [5, 61, 63, 67, 69]. Still, others do not exclude concomitant involvement of the peripheral and central vestibular systems [64, 68]. Vertebral artery compression leading to hemodynamic ischemic depolarization of the labyrinth could theoretically result in asymmetric excitation of the neurons and inner ear cells (especially in the compressed VA side) causing transient "irritative" nystagmus [5]. Nystagmus waveform and tinnitus side corroborate this theory in some cases [5, 65, 71]. Alternatively, transient inferior cerebellar hypoperfusion could promote asymmetrical disinhibition of the vestibular nuclei [66, 72]. Cerebral blood flow scintigraphy performed in one patient with RVAS showed decreased blood flow in the lower portion of the left cerebellar hemisphere, suggesting the presence of hemodynamic compromise in that area [73].

Management of RVAS remains controversial. Anticoagulation, endovascular stenting or conservative management with an antiplatelet agent have all been considered as treatment options [63, 67, 68]. A small case series from the 1990s reported that 50% of patients treated conservatively went on to develop neurologic deficits; accordingly, surgical therapy including decompression of VA and/or cervical fusion has been recommended as the treatment of choice [7, 64, 69]. More recently, a study with 21 RVAS patients showed a favorable long-term outcome in the conservative treatment group [66].

Conclusion

When observing a patient with nystagmus and/or vertigo, positional testing can be a valuable addition to the clinical assessment. In addition to the normal sitting position with the head upright, positional/positioning maneuvers that bring the head into a supine, head-hanging and forward bending position shoud be examined. While in these positions, head rotation to the sides should also be evaluated as well. Preferentially, testing is done with and without ocular fixation, since asymptomatic healthy individuals may show slow velocity positional nystagmus only in dark, as opposed to pathological states which usually display positional nystagmus and/or vertigo in light and dark conditions. Persistent nystagmus without vertigo and intense short-lasting vertigo and/or vomiting with slight or no nystagmus are two common presentations of central positional dizziness requiring urgent imaging, preferentially an MRI study. Vertigo and nystagmus that manifest strictly on head rotation can be a harbinger of impending vertebral artery occlusion. Dynamic angiography demonstrates vertebral artery compression on head rotation in these cases. Treatment options include surgery, endovascular stenting and oral anticoagulation.

References

[1] Bertholon P, Tringali S, Faye MB, Antoine JC, Martin C. Prospective study of positional nystagmus in 100 consecutive patients. *Ann Otol Rhinol Laryngol.* 2006 Aug;115(8):587-94.

[2] Buttner-Ennever JA. A review of otolith pathways to brainstem and cerebellum. *Ann N Y Acad Sci.* 1999 May 28;871:51-64.

[3] Glasauer S, Dieterich M, Brandt T. Central positional nystagmus simulated by a mathematical ocular motor model of otolith-dependent modification of Listing's plane. *J Neurophysiol.* 2001 Oct;86(4):1546-54.

[4] Watson P, Barber HO, Deck J, Terbrugge K. Positional vertigo and nystagmus of central origin. *Can J Neurol Sci.* 1981 May;8(2):133-7.

[5] Marti S, Hegemann S, von Budingen HC, Baumgartner RW, Straumann D. Rotational vertebral artery syndrome: 3D kinematics of nystagmus suggest bilateral labyrinthine dysfunction. *J Neurol.* 2008 May;255(5):663-7.

[6] Buttner U, Helmchen C, Brandt T. Diagnostic criteria for central versus peripheral positioning nystagmus and vertigo: a review. *Acta Otolaryngol.* 1999 Jan;119(1):1-5.

[7] Kuether TA, Nesbit GM, Clark WM, Barnwell SL. Rotational vertebral artery occlusion: a mechanism of vertebrobasilar insufficiency. *Neurosurgery.* 1997 Aug;41(2):427-32; discussion 32-3.

[8] Kim HA, Yi HA, Lee H. Apogeotropic central positional nystagmus as a sole sign of nodular infarction. *Neurol Sci.* 2012 Oct;33(5):1189-91.

[9] Drachman DA, Diamond ER, Hart CW. Posturally-evoked vomiting; Association with posterior fossa lesions. *Ann Otol Rhinol Laryngol.* 1977 Jan-Feb;86(1 Pt 1):97-101.

[10] Katsarkas A. Vestibular and oculomotor disturbances in pathology of the fourth ventricle. *Laryngoscope.* 1981 Jan;91(1):71-7.

[11] Kattah JC, Gujrati M. Familial positional downbeat nystagmus and cerebellar ataxia: clinical and pathologic findings. *Ann N Y Acad Sci.* 2005 Apr;1039:540-3.

[12] Lee JY, Lee WW, Kim JS, Kim HJ, Kim JK, Jeon BS. Perverted head-shaking and positional downbeat nystagmus in patients with multiple system atrophy. *Mov Disord.* 2009 Jul 15;24(9):1290-5.

[13] Gregorius FK, Crandall PH, Baloh RW. Positional vertigo with cerebellar astrocytoma. *Surg Neurol.* 1976 Nov;6(5):283-6.

[14] von Brevern M, Zeise D, Neuhauser H, Clarke AH, Lempert T. Acute migrainous vertigo: clinical and oculographic findings. *Brain.* 2005 Feb;128(Pt 2):365-74.

[15] Cawthorne T, Hinchcliffe R. Positional nystagmus of the central type as evidence of subtentorial metastases. *Brain.* 1961 Sep;84:415-26.

[16] Baloh RW, Spooner JW. Downbeat nystagmus: a type of central vestibular nystagmus. *Neurology.* 1981 Mar;31(3):304-10.

[17] Bertholon P, Bronstein AM, Davies RA, Rudge P, Thilo KV. Positional down beating nystagmus in 50 patients: cerebellar disorders and possible anterior semicircular canalithiasis. *J Neurol Neurosurg Psychiatry.* 2002 Mar;72(3):366-72.

[18] Walker MF, Tian J, Shan X, Ying H, Tamargo RJ, Zee DS. Enhancement of the Bias Component of Downbeat Nystagmus after Lesions of the Nodulus and Uvula. Annals of the New York Academy of Sciences. 2009;1164(1):482-5.

[19] Nylen C. The oto-neurological diagnosis of tumors of the brain. *Acta Otolaryngol.* 1939; 33 (suppl):1-151.

[20] Harrison MS, Ozsahinoglu C. Positional vertigo: aetiology and clinical significance. *Brain.* 1972;95(2):369-72.

[21] Thomsen J, Zilstorff K, Johnsen NJ. Positional nystagmus of the persistent type. *ORL J Otorhinolaryngol Relat Spec. 1978*;40(2):86-91.

[22] Brandt T. Positional and positioning vertigo and nystagmus. *J Neurol Sci.* 1990 Jan;95(1):3-28.

[23] Williams LG, Brimage P, Lechner C, Taylor RL, Masters L, Welgampola MS. Lhermitte-Duclos disease presenting with atypical positional nystagmus. *J Clin Neurosci.* 2014 May 16.

[24] Allen G, Fernandez C. Experimental observations in postural nystagmus. I. Extensive lesions in posterior vermis of the cerebellum. *Acta Otolaryngol.* 1960 Jan-Feb;51:2-14.

[25] Fernandez C, Alzate R, Lindsay JR. Experimental observations on postural nystagmus. II. Lesions of the nodulus. *Ann Otol Rhinol Laryngol.* 1960 Mar;69:94-114.

[26] Nam J, Kim S, Huh Y, Kim JS. Ageotropic central positional nystagmus in nodular infarction. *Neurology.* 2009 Oct 6;73(14):1163.

[27] Aschan G, Ekvall L, Grant G. Nystagmus Following Stimulation in the Central Vestibular Pathways Using Permanently Implanted Electrodes. *Acta Otolaryngol Suppl.* 1963;192:SUPPL 192:63+.

[28] Yee RD, Baloh RW, Honrubia V. Episodic vertical oscillopsia and downbeat nystagmus in a Chiari malformation. *Arch Ophthalmol.* 1984 May;102(5):723-5.

[29] Polensek SH, Tusa RJ. Nystagmus during attacks of vestibular migraine: an aid in diagnosis. *Audiol Neurootol.* 2010;15(4):241-6.

[30] Anderson T, Luxon L, Quinn N, Daniel S, Marsden CD, Bronstein A. Oculomotor function in multiple system atrophy: clinical and laboratory features in 30 patients. *Mov Disord.* 2008 May 15;23(7):977-84.

[31] Katsarkas A. Positional nystagmus of the "central type" as an early sign of multiple sclerosis. *J Otolaryngol.* 1982 Apr;11(2):91-3.

[32] Yu-Wai-Man P, Gorman G, Bateman DE, Leigh RJ, Chinnery PF. Vertigo and vestibular abnormalities in spinocerebellar ataxia type 6. *J Neurol.* 2009 Jan;256(1):78-82.

[33] Sunami K, Tochino R, Zushi T, Yamamoto H, Tokuhara Y, Iguchi H, et al. Positional and positioning nystagmus in healthy subjects under videonystagmoscopy. *Acta Otolaryngol Suppl.* 2004 Oct(554):35-7.

[34] Bisdorff AR, Sancovic S, Debatisse D, Bentley C, Gresty MA, Bronstein AM. Positional nystagmus in the dark in normal subjects. *Neuroophthalmology.* 2000;24(1):283-90.

[35] Mulch G, Lewitzki W. Spontaneous and positional nystagmus in healthy persons demonstrated only by electronystagmography: physiological spontaneous nystagmus or "functional scar"? *Arch Otorhinolaryngol.* 1977 Apr 27;215(2):135-45.

[36] Daniel MM, Lionel Z, Robert JP. Humans use internal models to estimate gravity and linear acceleration. *Nature.* 1999;398(6728):615-8.

[37] Sakata E, Ohtsu K, Shimura H, Sakai S. Positional nystagmus of benign paroxysmal type (BPPN) due to cerebellar vermis lesions. Pseudo-BPPN. *Auris Nasus Larynx.* 1987;14(1):17-21.

[38] Imai T, Horii A, Takeda N, Kitahara T, Higashi-Shingai K, Inohara H. A case of apogeotropic nystagmus with brainstem lesion: An implication for mechanism of central apogeotropic nystagmus. *Auris Nasus Larynx.* 2010 Dec;37(6):742-6.

[39] Anagnostou E, Varaki K, Anastasopoulos D. A minute demyelinating lesion causing acute positional vertigo. *J Neurol Sci.* 2008 Mar 15;266(1-2):187-9.

[40] Arbusow V, Strupp M, Brandt T. Amiodarone-induced severe prolonged head-positional vertigo and vomiting. *Neurology.* 1998 Sep;51(3):917.

[41] Lea J, Lechner C, Halmagyi GM, Welgampola MS. Not so benign positional vertigo: paroxysmal downbeat nystagmus from a superior cerebellar peduncle neoplasm. *Otol Neurotol.* 2014 Jul;35(6):e204-5.

[42] Büttner U, Brandt T, Helmchen C. The direction of nystagmus is important for the diagnosis of central paroxysmal positioning nystagmus (cPPV). *Neuro-Ophthalmology.* 1999 2014/07/19;21(2):97-104.

[43] Bassani R, Della Torre S. Positional nystagmus reversing from geotropic to apogeotropic: a new central vestibular syndrome. *J Neurol.* 2011 Feb;258(2):313-5.

[44] Anagnostou E, Mandellos D, Limbitaki G, Papadimitriou A, Anastasopoulos D. Positional nystagmus and vertigo due to a solitary brachium conjunctivum plaque. *J Neurol Neurosurg Psychiatry.* 2006 Jun;77(6):790-2.

[45] Kattah JC, Kolsky MP, Luessenhop AJ. Positional vertigo and the cerebellar vermis. *Neurology.* 1984 Apr;34(4):527-9.

[46] Saber Tehrani AS, Kattah JC, Mantokoudis G, Pula JH, Nair D, Blitz A, et al. Small strokes causing severe vertigo: Frequency of false-negative MRIs and nonlacunar mechanisms. *Neurology.* 2014 Jul 8;83(2):169-73.

[47] Choi SY, Park SH, Kim HJ, Kim JS. Paraneoplastic downbeat nystagmus associated with cerebellar hypermetabolism especially in the nodulus. *J Neurol Sci.* 2014 Aug 15;343(1-2):187-91.

[48] Helmchen C, Gottschalk S, Sander T, Trillenberg P, Rambold H, Sprenger A. Beneficial effects of 3,4-diaminopyridine on positioning downbeat nystagmus in a circumscribed uvulo-nodular lesion. *J Neurol.* 2007 Aug;254(8):1126-8.

[49] Choi JY, Park YM, Woo YS, Kim SU, Jung JM, Kwon DY. Perverted head-shaking and positional downbeat nystagmus in pregabalin intoxication. *J Neurol Sci.* 2014 Feb 15;337(1-2):243-4.

[50] Pollak L, Klein C, Rabey JM, Reichenthal E. Posturally evoked vomiting without nystagmus in a patient with Arnold-Chiari malformation. *J Neurol Neurosurg Psychiatry.* 2001 Sep;71(3):414-5.

[51] Jen JC, Yue Q, Karrim J, Nelson SF, Baloh RW. Spinocerebellar ataxia type 6 with positional vertigo and acetazolamide responsive episodic ataxia. *J Neurol Neurosurg Psychiatry.* 1998 Oct;65(4):565-8.

[52] Kremmyda O, Zwergal A, la Fougere C, Brandt T, Jahn K, Strupp M. 4-Aminopyridine suppresses positional nystagmus caused by cerebellar vermis lesion. *J Neurol.* 2013 Jan;260(1):321-3.

[53] Kearsley JH, Johnson P, Halmagyi GM. Paraneoplastic cerebellar disease. Remission with excision of the primary tumor. *Arch Neurol.* 1985 Dec;42(12):1208-10.

[54] Eggers SD, Pittock SJ, Shepard NT, Habermann TM, Neff BA, Klebig RR. Positional periodic alternating vertical nystagmus with PCA-Tr antibodies in Hodgkin lymphoma. *Neurology.* 2012 May 29;78(22):1800-2.

[55] Barber HO. Positional nystagmus. *Otolaryngol Head Neck Surg.* 1984 Dec;92(6):649-55.

[56] Lechner C, Taylor RL, Todd C, Macdougall H, Yavor R, Halmagyi GM, et al. Causes and characteristics of horizontal positional nystagmus. *J Neurol.* 2014 May;261(5):1009-17.

[57] Fetter M, Haslwanter T, Bork M, Dichgans J. New insights into positional alcohol nystagmus using three-dimensional eye-movement analysis. *Ann Neurol.* 1999 Feb;45(2):216-23.

[58] Aschan G, Stahle J. Nystagmus in Meniere's disease during attacks; a nystagmographical study. *Acta Otolaryngol.* 1957 Mar;47(3):189-201.

[59] Taylor RL, Chen L, Lechner C, Aw ST, Welgampola MS. Vestibular schwannoma mimicking horizontal cupulolithiasis. *J Clin Neurosci.* 2013 Aug;20(8):1170-3.

[60] Lee SH, Kim JS. Benign paroxysmal positional vertigo. *J Clin Neurol.* 2010 Jun;6(2):51-63.

[61] Lu DC, Zador Z, Mummaneni PV, Lawton MT. Rotational vertebral artery occlusion-series of 9 cases. *Neurosurgery.* 2010 Oct;67(4):1066-72; discussion 72.

[62] Toole JF, Tucker SH. Influence of head position upon cerebral circulation. Studies on blood flow in cadavers. *Arch Neurol.* 1960 Jun;2:616-23.

[63] Kim HA, Yi HA, Lee CY, Lee H. Origin of isolated vertigo in rotational vertebral artery syndrome. *Neurol Sci.* 2011 Dec;32(6):1203-7.

[64] Choi KD, Shin HY, Kim JS, Kim SH, Kwon OK, Koo JW, et al. Rotational vertebral artery syndrome: oculographic analysis of nystagmus. *Neurology.* 2005 Oct 25;65(8):1287-90.

[65] Strupp M, Planck JH, Arbusow V, Steiger HJ, Bruckmann H, Brandt T. Rotational vertebral artery occlusion syndrome with vertigo due to "labyrinthine excitation". *Neurology.* 2000 Mar 28;54(6):1376-9.

[66] Choi KD, Choi JH, Kim JS, Kim HJ, Kim MJ, Lee TH, et al. Rotational vertebral artery occlusion: mechanisms and long-term outcome. *Stroke.* 2013 Jul;44(7):1817-24.

[67] Choi KH, Lee SH, Kim JM, Oh DS, Kim JT, Park MS, et al. Rotational vertebral artery syndrome in moyamoya disease: a sign of unilateral vertebral artery stenosis. *Clin Neurol Neurosurg.* 2013 Sep;115(9):1900-2.

[68] Park SH, Kim SJ, Seo JD, Kim DH, Choi JH, Choi KD, et al. Upbeat nystagmus during head rotation in rotational vertebral artery occlusion. *J Neurol.* 2014 Jun;261(6):1213-5.

[69] Rosengart A, Hedges TR, 3rd, Teal PA, DeWitt LD, Wu JK, Wolpert S, et al. Intermittent downbeat nystagmus due to vertebral artery compression. *Neurology.* 1993 Jan;43(1):216-8.

[70] Vilela MD, Goodkin R, Lundin DA, Newell DW. Rotational vertebrobasilar ischemia: hemodynamic assessment and surgical treatment. *Neurosurgery.* 2005;56(1):36-43; discussion -5.

[71] Cohen B, Suzuki JI, Bender MB. Eye Movements from Semicircular Canal Nerve Stimulation in the Cat. *Ann Otol Rhinol Laryngol.* 1964 Mar;73:153-69.

[72] Noh Y, Kwon OK, Kim HJ, Kim JS. Rotational vertebral artery syndrome due to compression of nondominant vertebral artery terminating in posterior inferior cerebellar artery. *J Neurol.* 2011 Oct;258(10):1775-80.

[73] Matsuyama T, Morimoto T, Sakaki T. Bow Hunter's stroke caused by a nondominant vertebral artery occlusion: case report. *Neurosurgery.* 1997 Dec;41(6):1393-5.

In: Eye Movement Disorders
Editor: Sloan L. Mills

ISBN: 978-1-63321-980-9

Chapter 4

The Treatment of Intermittent Exotropia in Childhood: A Long-Term Study

Elfriede Stangler-Zuschrott*
University Eye-Clinic Vienna emeritus,
Austrian Academy of Ophthalmology and Optometry, Vienna, Austria

Abstract

This study presents 124 children aged less than 15 years suffering from a temporary divergent squint when looking into the far distance. These children were treated and observed in an ophthalmologist's office over the past 35 years.

No evidence-based rules for treating intermittent divergent squints are found in the literature. The possibilities are: (1) Prescription of glasses, (2) Short-term occlusion of one eye against suppression, (3) Orthoptic exercises, (4) Prismatic correction of the squint over some years, (5) Surgery, and (6) Contact lenses in older and myopic children.

The aim of treatment is to establish a steady compensated exophoria with a latent angle as small as possible; in rare cases the result may be orthophoria.

* Corresponding author's email: e.stangler-zuschrott@aon.at.

The patients sample showed some specific characteristics: 44.5% started squinting in the 2nd and 3rd year of life, 76.6% had unilateral strabismus and suppression, but no severe amblyopia and - 67% had approximate emmetropia, which played a role in compliance with wearing glasses.

Most ophthalmologists prefer to wait and observe the child for some time; if the child's squint deteriorates, an operation will be proposed. The success of such operations is uncertain.

I adopted a conservative treatment approach starting with prisms. Unlike older children the younger children – aged less than 10 years – mostly accepted the glasses necessary to apply the press-on-prisms which correct the squint angle for distance. After a short time, the eye position fixing near objects relaxes and the children had almost the same squint deviation for near and distant fixation. Therefore the diagnosis was "pseudodivergence excess" in almost all the children, only two had convergence insufficiency and two others needed bifocals. In periodical controls, the prisms were adapted to the current eye position. In this way, - in spite of squint – fusion was trained throughout the day and suppression eliminated. Step-by-step the squint angle decreased, with a reduction of on average 13Δ, and finally, after average 4.3 years the prisms could be removed. The longer the time of prism-treatment, the more constant was the result, even after years. This method is recommended only for children with a squint deviation of up to 10°. More severe squints require surgery; but the results are better after preparation of the binocular functions by prisms. A small postoperative divergence can be treated again with prisms or with contact lenses in cases of myopia.

The therapy should be started as soon as possible after the onset of the squint, as the recovery time will be less. Parents should be warned that treatment takes a long time. However, treatment is safe and results in good sensorial preconditions for adult life.

Introduction

Children with a periodic divergent squint are a heterogeneous group – and their treatment is not evidence-based. Therefore, I would like to share the experiences I have gained over the past 35 years.

A child closing one eye in bright sunshine is considered the typical first behavioral symptom of a divergent squint. Probably the child experiences double vision and unlike an adult can quickly adjust to normal vision by suppressing the deviating eye. Thus, we cannot differentiate in childhood between decompensating exophoria and intermittent exotropia; the first results in diplopia, the second in suppression or, later on, other sensorial adaptations.

Clinical features are a child tired, feeling bored or sick, not fixing a certain object, and suddenly turning one eye outwards, which the child is able to correct immediately. One eye drifts outwards only when looking into the far distance while not fixing a near object. With time, the squint phases become longer and more frequent and a stage is reached when the parents seek treatment.

Pathophysiology

The dynamics underlying an intermittent divergent strabismus are unknown. Most ophthalmologists suppose an abnormal "position of rest" of the eye-balls in the divergent orbits. With effort the eyes can be forced to converge to a normal straight position with binocular functions. Thus, the divergence is overcome by "convergence excess". [1] Another theory designates the turning out of one eye as "divergence excess [2], assuming that an active monocular divergence is possible. As yet, no center for divergence functions has been located in the brain; therefore, some ophthalmologists explain a divergent position of the eyes by passive relaxation into the "position of rest" [3]. The study of my patient cohort aimed to give new insights.

The Patients

The study included 124 patients aged up to 15 years who were registered at my office and diagnosed with intermittent exotropia. Not included were patients showing organic defects of the eyes, hypothyreosis, mental disability, cerebral palsy, hydrocephalus, premature birth, eye muscle palsies and consecutive divergence, e.g. after surgical intervention to correct convergence.

Some interesting observations were made upon examination of the whole sample:

- Heredity: 20.8% of the children had a family history of intermittent exotropia, assuming the information provided by the children's parents was complete.

- Age at the onset of squint (Figure 1): 44.5% of the children started to squint in their 2nd or 3rd year of life, corresponding to the literature.
- Laterality: 76.6% of the children had an unilateral strabismus, the ratio of right to left eye deviation was 52 : 43. However, none of the patients had a severe amblyopia, only two showed a reduced unilateral visual acuity of 0.5. These patients were treated by short-term occlusion.
- Refraction: The eyes of 120 children were cycloplegically refracted using Lindner's retinoscopy [4]. Surprisingly, 67.5% were found to have approximate emmetropia, i.e., a range between -0.5 D and +0.75 D spherical equivalent (Table 1). No human has exactly 0 D.

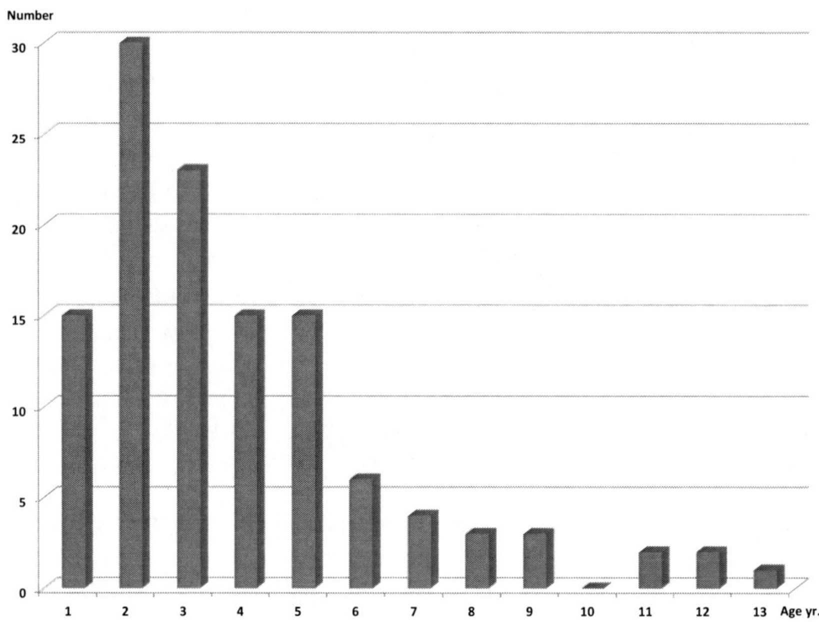

Figure 1. Age at the onset of squint.

A recent study [5] reported that only 25% of the not squinting children aged 2-3 years examined were emmetropic, in contrast to my study, where 71.8% of the children of the same age with intermittent divergent squint were emmetropic. (Table 2). In textbooks [6] the normal refraction of children at this age is assumed to be +2.0 D. The prevailing emmetropia amongst my patient cohort is key to understanding why these children refused to wear glasses and it was so difficult to use prism therapy with them. 32.5% of my patients needed fully correcting glasses of the refractive error, exceptionally in hyperopic cases 0.5 D were subtracted.

Table 1. Refraction error (120 cases)

	Number	
Emmetropia	81	-
Hyperopia	21	1-2 D
Hyperopia	5	>2 D
Anisometropia	3	>1 D
Myopia	5	>1 D
Astigmatism	5	>1 D

Table 2. Age and refraction error (120 cases)

	Number	Emmetropia
Age 2-3 yrs	64	46 = 71,8%
Age 4-15 yrs	56	35 = 62,5%
Total	120	81 = **67,5%**

Treatment Method and Results

1. Wait and Observe

Strabismus remains stable for years in some children, but in others the phases of deviation become more frequent and longer. There is an unwritten rule that operation is appropriate if the squinting period exceeds half the time of the child's vigil. The rational is to prevent the development of a steady divergent strabismus and consequent sensorial adaptations. Most ophthalmologists attempt to resolve squints by surgery.

The question arises whether a spontaneous improvement with a change to exophoria is possible. Hiles [7] found that 31 of 48 patients decreased their deviation by an average of 18Δ after a mean of 11.7 years, but normalization was not achieved.

Results of the Study

Three children with an intermittent squint in their 2nd year of life were orthophoric six months later without having received any treatment. Similar spontaneous remissions were never observed in older patients.

2. Glasses

The prescription of glasses depends on the kind of refraction error and, whether or not the child squints. Children who squint – convergent or divergent – require fully correcting glasses, even with low diopters. This is because convergence, accommodation and fusion form a sensitive control system of binocularity; these components influence each other. Even a slight accommodative relaxation with glasses of only +0.5 D may increase the fusion range [8] and relieve exophoric patients of asthenopic complaints. The recommendation in the literature [9] is to prescribe minus-lenses to overcome the divergence by activating the accommodative convergence. This method does not seem to be physiologic and may overstrain the accommodative power. In a recent study [10] children with intermittent exotropia were found to have a reduced accommodative amplitude compared with controls.

Results of the Study

Eight patients, aged between 4 and 13 years were treated with glasses alone; one had myopia of -4 D, the others a refraction error with a maximum of +1.5 D and glasses up to +1.0 D. Only one child refused to wear glasses. After 0.5 to 6 years' observation five patients reduced their squint angle from -25Δ to orthophoria, and the others had at least well compensated exophoria.

3. Occlusion

Occlusion seems to work against suppression of a deviating eye, but at the same time interrupts the fusion present at near fixation. One should consider that suppression of the squinting eye is produced binocularly and only occurs in those moments when the eye is in an anatomical outward-position; [11] therefore, elimination is only possible in this state by prismatic correction of the squint angle.

Occlusion of the master eye is indicated to treat amblyopia or deep-rooted laterality. The occlusion film, fixed on the glass of the dominant eye, should be translucent and reduce the vision to an acuity of 0.1. Light impermeable foils could also be used, but only for a few hours a day.

Results of the Study

Two patients of pre-school age eliminated their squint within a few months.

4. Orthoptic Exercises

Orthoptists are obligated to give patients orthoptic exercises with the aim of improving the fusion depth, activating the convergence and eliminating suppression. Unfortunately, the exercises are time consuming.

Results of the Study

The control checkup of 13 patients after training showed more power to compensate the deviation, but the squint angle in general was the same as before.

5. Contact Lenses

In my experience, myopic patients who wear hard contact lenses (CL) reduce their squint angle. This is because more effort is needed for accommodation in eyes with CL. Another factor may be that the optical imaging in the periphery of the visual field is better with CL than with glasses. The peripheral visual perception is dominant over the central one when looking into the distance.

Result of the Study

The benefit of hard CL seen in two of my myopic patients:

Case 1: Girl, father squinting divergent
Age 14 yrs: Refraction: RE -5.75 +0.75x LE -6.5 +0.75x
Decompensating exophoria, sometimes diplopia
Squint angle distance (F) -35Δ, near (N) -40Δ
Age 18 yrs: Fitting of hard CL resulting in → exophoria
Age 41 yrs: After wearing the CL since 23 yrs: F = N exophoria,
Latent angle F = N -14Δ

Case 2: Girl

Age 12 yrs: Refraction: RE -2.5s, LE -1.25s
Intermittent divergent squint, angle F -30Δ, N -4Δ

Age 17 yrs: wearing CL, squint angle F -4Δ, N -2Δ

6. Long-Term Wearing of Prisms without Operation (19 Patients)

6.1. Background

In 1967, French researchers [12, 13] found that continuously wearing prisms corrected squint deviations; the prisms were progressively reduced and no operations were needed if the angle did not exceed 8° or 10°.

Press-on prisms have been available in Austria since 1970 and have been used at the 1. University Eye Clinic in Vienna with success one year before a squint operation [14].

Long-term observations of numerous patients have revealed that – in some cases-- there is a spontaneous reduction of the deviation or a consecutive divergence some years after an operation. Furthermore many patients, operated in early childhood, squinting again when adult. This raises the question of whether the ophthalmologists are performing too many operations on children of too young an age. Is there another therapeutic way? My first series of cases where patients were treated only with prismatic glasses was published in 1998 [15]. Intermittent divergent cases were not included in that study.

6.2. Guidelines for Fitting Prisms

The strength of the prisms base in (-Δ) is determined by the alternating cover-test at both distances, far and near.[16] Once the prisms fit, no movement should occur at any distance. At this point the Bagolini test is positive in many cases. Both eyes should be controlled by the unilateral cover-test; if a manifest deviation is evident, the prism power is insufficient. Press-ons should be used at the start of treatment, 20Δ maximum for each eye. The prisms should be applied to both eyes with the stronger one on the dominant eye against suppression. The difference between the right and left eye should not exceed 10Δ.

Shortly after the first application of the prisms the eye position for near fixation relaxes from parallel to divergent; now the same prismatic power fits for both distances, the "pseudo-divergence-excess" type of squint has changed into a basic type. Check the prisms every 2nd month and be careful not to overlook the development of an amblyopia behind the prisms, which may be caused by a microtropia, not by the prisms per se. For cosmetic reasons school children are given total or partially correcting prismatic glasses without or with thin press-ons.

6.3. Guidelines for Reducing the Prisms

If the alternating cover-test shows a movement from the nasal to temporal side, the prisms are overcorrecting and need to be reduced. If the prisms seem to be correct, a trial is possible: Apply a press-on of low power base out to one prismatic glass and let the patient wait for half an hour; possibly, in this time the child will stabilize a new eye position and reduced prisms can be ordered.

After different intervals of time the squint deviation changes slowly to a straight direction. The best possible result is orthophoria with good stereo-acuity. Most of my patients showed at least a slight and well compensated exophoria without wearing prismatic glasses.

6.4. Results of the Study (19 Patients)

Prismatic glasses were unsuccessful in two of the patients who wore (?) them for 5 years without any improvement. However, 17 patients had the staying power to finish the treatment and showed improvement.

For example (figure 2):

Case 3: Boy, onset of squint at age 3 yrs, deteriorating, Parents refused an operation

Age 7 yrs:	Intermittent exotropia LE, angle F = N -12Δ
	Refraction: RE +0.75s LE +0.75 +0.25x,
	VA: RE = LE 1.0
	Prisms: -12Δ distributed to both eyes
Age 8 yrs:	Prisms: -18Δ
Age 9-10 yrs:	Slow decrease to -10Δ
Age 11-15 yrs:	Decrease to -4Δ, prismatic glasses stop
Age 22:	Well compensated exophoria -6Δ, no complaints

To give a clearer overview, the sample of patients was divided into two groups according to their visual impairment estimated:

Group 1: Onset of squint at an early age with subsequent deterioration.

Group 2: Onset of squint at 4 years or older, decompensating only when tired, after a cover-test, occlusion or when excited.

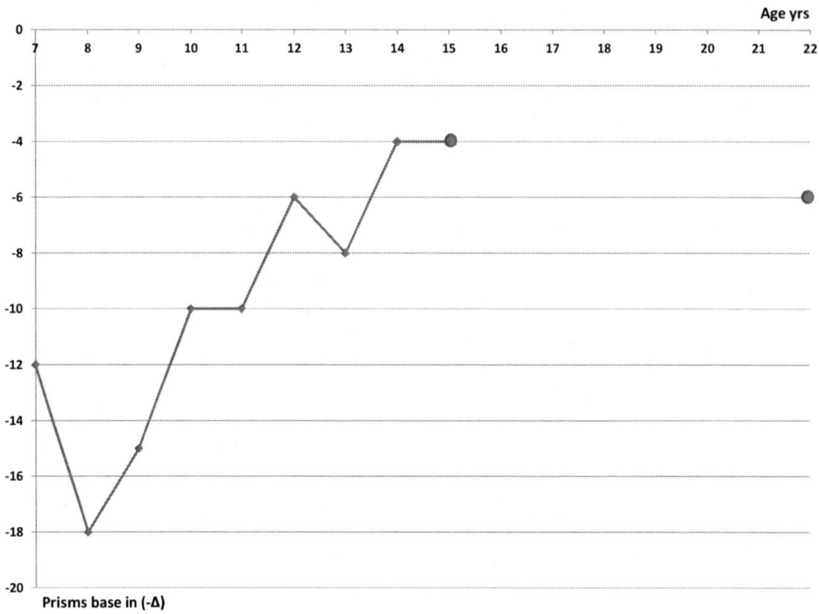

Figure 2. The fluctuations of the squint angle of case 3 during the prism treatment.

Table 3. Prism therapy alone (Group 1)

Name	C.L.	M.K.	W.M.	H.A.	K.M.	M-H.F.	W.C.	T.J.	K.J.	*av.*
Onset of squint										
age yr.	1	1	1	2	3	3	3	4	5	***2.6***
Start prisms										
age yr.	4	6	8	4	5	7	8	5	7	***6.0***
Δ	-12	-10	-20	-25	-22	-12	-18	-17	-20	***-17.3***
Final result										
age yr.	8	7	12	11	10	14.5	15	12	13	***11.4***
phoria Δ, no tropia	0	-6	-4	0	-16	-4	0	-5	-2	***-4.1***
Later findings										
age yr.	13				13	22	19		21	***17.6***
phoria Δ	-2				-4	-6	-10		0	***-4.4***
Duration of prism treatment yr.	4	1	4	7	5	7.5	7	7	6	***5.4***

Comment on group 1:

Prismatic treatment was initiated in most cases with a mean delay of 3.4 years; deviation was between 10 and 25 Δ base in, average 17.3Δ ; both, the time of onset and the degree of squint seemed to influence the time required to correct the squint (1-7.5 yrs, average 4.5 yrs). Every patient showed a remarkable reduction of the squint angle, average 13.2Δ, which remained constant after some years.

Comment on group 2:

The results for group 2 were more optimistic. These older children were treated with less delay, mean 1.8 yr; wearing of prisms lasted 0.5 - 8 yrs, average 3.1 yrs. The reduction of the angle was - similar to group 1 –an average of 13Δ. This seems to be the limit for improvement with the help of prisms. The two children who wore the prisms for the longest time had the worst starting positions -the largest squint angle or the longest delay of treatment.

Table 4. Prism therapy alone (Group 2)

Name	P.F.	M.S.	L.C.	B.T.	W.C.	G.M.	St.D.	St.L.	***av.***
Onset of squint									
age yr.	4	4	4	4.5	5	6	7	8	***5.3***
Start prisms									
age yr.	6	6	8	5	7	7	8	9	***7.0***
Δ	-15	-30	-20	-16	-20	-12	-20	-20	***-19.1***
Final result									
age yr.	6.5	11	16	6	9	10	10.5	12	***10.1***
phoria Δ, no tropia	-3	-14	-6	-2	-6	-6	-12	0	***-6.1***
Later findings									
age yr.		11	16			13			***13.3***
phoria Δ		-14	-12			0			***-8.7***
Duration of prism treatment yr.	0.5	5	8	1	2	3	2.5	3	***3.1***

7. Operation and Prisms Combined (20 Patients)

The sample was divided into two groups using the same criteria as above. Example from group 1, the more complicated group (figure 3).

Case 4: Boy, squint onset 1st year of life, convergence was trained at home.

Age 4 yrs: Squint angle F -24Δ, N -12Δ, refraction: RE +0.75s LE +0.5+0.25x

VA: RE = LE 1.0, first prisms: -12Δ each eye

Age 5 yrs: Prisms -35Δ distributed to both eyes

Age 6 yrs: Operation: LE Recession rect.ext. 5.5mm, resection rect. int. 4 mm

After the operation: angle F +8Δ, N 0Δ, prismatic correction and alternating occlusion were done, yet the angle increased up to +20Δ (diplopiaphobia). After 4 weeks the eye position was stable with +6Δ, no more occlusion was done, 2 months later the prisms were removed.

Age 9 yrs: Decompensating exophoria was again corrected with prisms up to -10Δ, decreasing to -3Δ.

Age 16 yrs: Glasses no longer required.

Age 18 yrs: orthophoria

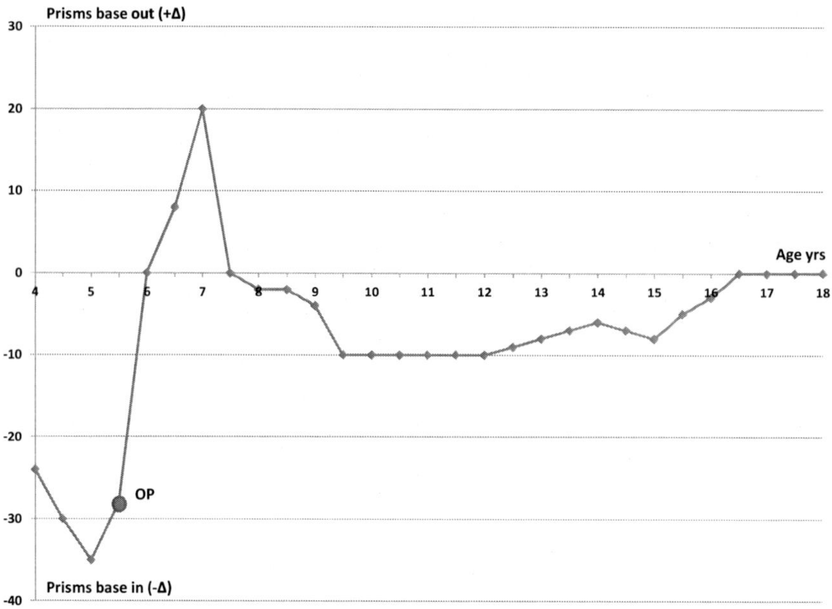

Figure 3. The fluctuations of the squint angle of case 4 during the prism treatment.

The Outcome of the Operated Group 1 (Table 5)

The initial squint angle was an average of -28.8Δ. In spite of the good operation results, in most cases the divergent position recurred within a few months of the operation and prisms were prescribed again. The patients who had the second prismatic correction seemed to have more stable long-term results. Only the one patient with the largest deviation needed a second operation. Example from group 2 (Figure 4):

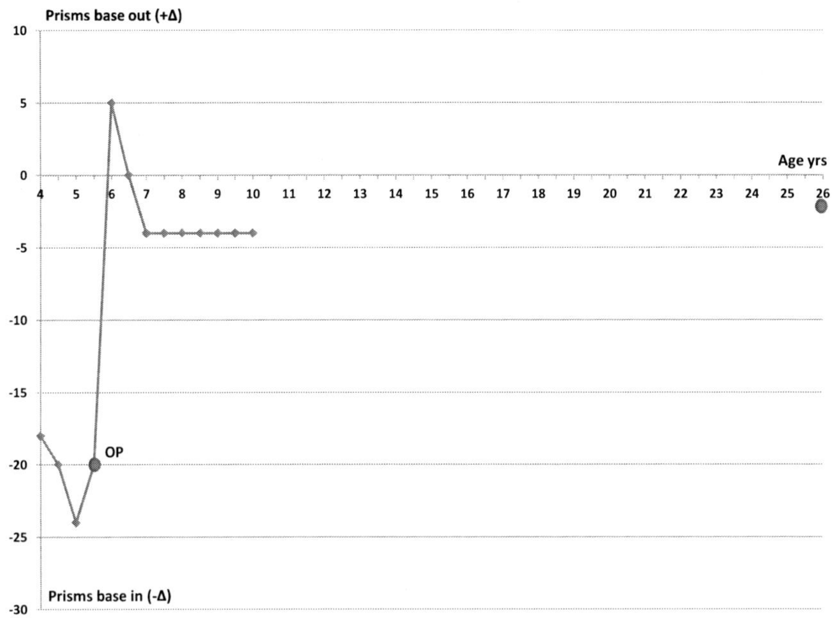

Figure 4. The fluctuations of the squint angle of case 5 during the prism treatment.

Table 5. Prism therapy + operation (Group1)

Name	B.C.	H.P.	Sch.C.	R.P.	E.M.	H.M.	K.C.	W.K.	Qu.H	H.I.	*av.*
Onset of squint											
age yr.	1	1	1	1	1.5	1.5	2	2	2	3	***1.6***
Start prisms											
age yr.	4	4	5	8	5	3	3	4	2	10	***4.8***
Δ	-40	-24	-25 Bifo	-35	-15	-25	-45	-30	-25	-20	***-28.8***
Operation											
age yr.	5	5.5	6	8.5	7	7	4	7	6	11	***6.7***
Result angle Δ	-6	0/+8	-4	-6	0	0	0	0	0	0	***-1.8***
Again prims											
age yr.		6/7	6.5			8	4.5	8	8		***7.0***
Δ		+20/-10	-15			-12	-35	-16	-15		***-18.6***
2. Operation											
age yr.							9				
Result angle Δ							0				
Final result											
age yr.	11	16	11	9	7	8	9	8	10	12	***10.1***
phoria Δ, no tropia	-8	-3	-6 Bifo	-18	0	-12	0	-16	-8	-4	***-7.7***
Later findings											
age yr.	30	18		19	9	17	16		21	18	***18.5***
phoria Δ	-3 CL	0		-16	0	-10	-8		-8 CL	-12	***-7.7***
Duration of prism treatment yr.	1	12	6	1	2	5	6	4	8	1	***4.6***

Case 5: Male

Age 4 years: divergence of right eye recently noticed. Refraction: RE -0.5+0.75x, LE -0.25+0.5x, VA RE = LE 1.0, RE suppression tendency

Age 4.5 yrs: First prisms: RE -5Δ, LE -12Δ, increasing to RE -8Δ, LE -15Δ

Age 6 yrs : Operation: RE Recession rect. ext. 4mm, resection rect. int. 3.5 mm

Result: 0Δ, stereopsis. 2 weeks later convergence +5Δ, prisms for 1 month

Age 10 yrs: Myopia is developing, exophoria -4Δ

Age 26 yrs: Exophoria -2Δ, contact lenses, no complaints

Table 6. Prism therapy + operation (Group 2)

Name	H.M.	L.O.	St.V.	G.T.	K.T.	Y.Y.	K.Th.	M.F.	St.M.	W.K.	***av.***
Onset of squint											
age yr.	2	2	2	4	4	4	5	5	5	8	***4.1***
Start prisms											
age yr.	5	4	4	4	5.5	4.5	6	5	5	8.5	***5.2***
Δ	-30	-22	-25	-20	-25	-35	-20	-15	-25	-22	***-23.9***
Operation											
age yr.	5.5	5	6	5.5	6	5.5	9	8	6	10	***6.7***
Result angle Δ	0	0	0	0	-10	0	-2	2	0	0	***-1.0***
Again prims											
age yr.	6	5.5	7	5.6							***6.0***
Δ	-6	-18	-16	5							***-8.8***
Final result											
age yr.	8	8	8	6	7	6	9.5	11	7	10.5	***8.1***
phoria Δ, no tropia	-4	-16	-10	-4	-10	0 Bifo	-12	-8	-2	-2	***-7.6***
Later findings											
age yr.		10	27	26	11	15	22	16	10	12	***16.6***
phoria Δ		-16	-8 CL	-2	-14	0 Bifo	-16	-10	-16	-4	***-11.1***
Duration of prism treatment yr.	3	4	4	1.6	0.5	1	3	3	1	1.5	***2.3***

The Outcome of the Operated Group 2 (Table 6)

The initial squint angle was a mean of 23.9Δ (smaller than in group 1), prisms were worn for an average 2.3 years (shorter than for group 1). Only 4 patients needed prisms again after surgery and, -no one needed a second operation. But the degree of the remaining exophoria, measured in the patients at an older age, was the highest among the four prism-treated groups.

8. No or Uncompleted Treatment (57 cases)

Asked for second opinion	33
Non-compliance, refusing glasses	12
Prism treatment not yet finished	5
Prism treatment broken off	7

Conclusion

1. The Practice

The aim of the study was to establish the best way to treat patients with intermittent exotropia. Sometimes this problem solves spontaneously without any treatment, but only before the age of 2.5 years. To observe a child and wait for longer is a waste of time in my experience. Considering the potential benefit, I would choose to prescribe glasses as a first step, regardless of the type of refraction error because sometimes glasses do help. As a next step I recommend fitting prisms. These stabilize the eyes in the divergent position, which seems paradoxical but in reality bifoveal perception is possible in this position; fusion is trained during the day with a simultaneous elimination of suppression. The prisms should correct the total deviation because complete relaxation of the eye position is necessary to prevent overacting convergence impulses that draw the divergent eyes inside again [1]. Orthoptic exercises for convergence are not advisable at this state of treatment. The child learns by the prisms that the divergence is the "normal" position. After some years binocular functions are established and become strong enough to maintain an almost straight eye position. This gentle and physiologic treatment is effective only for squint deviations up to 10°; more severe cases require an operation. There are many unfavorable reports in the literature [3 and 18] of high rates of recurrence after these operations. Surgery is an intervention which particularly disrupts the equilibrium between the eye pair -as can to be seen in case 4 reported here. Therefore, it is advisable to additionally treat patients with prisms before and, if necessary, after surgery.

Treatment of a child who squints should be started as soon as possible to shorten the time of recovery. Based on experience with my patient cohort, I believe, the longer the prismatic glasses are used, the more stable and lasting are the benefits. It seems to be important to have an as small as possible angle of exophoria at the end of the treatment. Modern working conditions that involve long periods of concentration on a computer screen are unfavorable for eyes. Many adults -who were operated in childhood – require further surgery because of asthenopic complaints and decompensating divergent squints.

The difficulties in implementing the prism method which are probably the reason why prisms are not the standard method of strabismology, are well-known: Compliance with the wearing of glasses, many years of treatment with periodical controls; the method is time consuming but safe. However, many parents of squinting children prefer the shorter surgical treatment without anything else.

2. The Theory

Some authors have postulated that divergent squints are caused by anatomical hindrances in the orbit. This may be right for extreme cases of divergence like Morbus Crouzon, but not for common cases of intermittent exotropia. If the "position of rest" can be normalized by prisms, the anatomy must be normal. The position of rest seems to be based on the tonic innervation of the eye muscles, tonic vergence, accommodative and fusional vergence.

Returning to refraction, the 67% of emmetropic patients. If hypermetropia of +2D is the common refraction in early childhood and babies have a distance of sight about 1m in daily life, an accommodative effort of 4 – 5 D and adequate convergence are necessary for clear binocular vision. In Donders' opinion [19], myopic babies may develop an exodeviation on the base of an underactive accommodation-convergence mechanism. My patients seemed to confirm this thesis.

I cannot exclude other concepts of squint origin, for example that active innervational impulses cause the turning out of one eye. I have seen a boy of 7 years who suddenly started to squint when his parents got divorced.

The chapter of intermitting divergence is not yet closed. More scientific investigations need to be done.

Acknowledgment

I would like to thank Elise Langdon-Neuner for copyediting the manuscript and Mag. Reinhard Müller for support in computer-technics.

References

[1] Wieser, D.; (1986) Die präoperative Prismenbehandlung bei intermittierender Exotropie. *Augenärztliche Fortbildung* 9, 33-39.

[2] Burian H.M.; (1966) Exodeviations: Their classification, diagnosis and treatment. *Amer. J. Ophthal.*, Serv. 3, 62, 1161-1166.

[3] Kaufmann H., Steffen H., Strabismus, 4th edition, *Georg Thieme Verlag*, Stuttgart, 2012.

[4] Lindner, K.; Die Bestimmung des Astigmatismus durch die Schattenprobe mit Cylindergläsern. S. Karger Verlag, Berlin 1927.

[5] Multi-ethnic pediatric eye disease study group. (2010) Prevalence of myopia and hyperopia in 6-72 month old African American and Hispanic children: the multi-ethnic pediatric eye desease study. *Ophthalmology*, 2010; 117(1):140-7.

[6] Lang J.; Strabismus 5th edition, Hans Huber Verlag, Bern, 2003.

[7] Hiles, Davies and Costenbader; (1968) cit. in Duke-Elder St; System of Ophthalmology, Vol. VI: Ocular Motility and Strabismus. Henry Kimpton, London 1973, page 630.

[8] Stangler-Zuschrott, E. (1981) Über die Verordnung von Brillen mit geringfügiger Korrektionswirkung. *Klin.Mbl.Augenheilk.*181, 493 – 495.

[9] Hugonnier,R.,Magnard, P. (1983) Schielen. In: Francois J, Hollwich F.: Augenheilkunde in Klinik und Praxis. Georg Thieme Verlag, Stuttgart, page 1174.

[10] Tejedor, J., Gutierrez, F.J. (2013) Accommodative amplitude in intermittent exotropia. In: Transactions oft he 36th ESA Meeting Sept. 4-7 Marseille, page 295. Ed. Olav H. Haugen, Bergen.

[11] Pratt-Johnson J, Tillson G. (2001) Management of Strabismus and Amblyopia. 2nd Edition, Thieme, Stuttgart. Page 129.

[12] Berard, P.V., Payan-Papera M. (1967): Les Prismes. *Bull. Soc. Ophthal. Fr.* 67, 581.

[13] Ravault, A.P., Bongrand, M., Bonamour G., (1972) The utilization of prisms in the treatment of divergent strabismus. In: Orhtoptics,

Proceedings of the 2nd international Orthoptic Congress, Amsterdam. Ed. Mein, et al., Excerpta Medica, Amsterdam.

[14] Stangler-Zuschrott E. (1980) Acht Jahre Prismenbehandlung des Strabismus convergens alternans. *Klin. Mbl. Augenheilk.* 177, 835-838

[15] Stangler-Zuschrott E. (1998): Long-term wearing of prisms – A conservative way to cure squint deviations in childhood? In: Advances in strabismology, proceedings of the 8th meeting of ISA, Maastricht. Ed. G. Lennerstrand, Aeolus Press, Buren, the Netherlands.

[16] Stangler-Zuschrott,E., (2012) Prismen zur Behandlung des Strabismus bei Kindern. Prisms in the treatment of infantile strabismus. *Spektrum Augenheilk.* 26, 230-235.

[17] Noorden G.K. Binocular Vision and Ocular Motility 5th Edition (1996).

[18] Gregersen, E., (1969) The polymorphous Exo Patient. *Acta Ophthalmologica* 47, 579-590.

[19] Lang, J. (1966) Zur Donders'schen Theorie des akkommodativen Schielens. *Ophthalmologica* 152, 453-460.

In: Eye Movement Disorders
Editor: Sloan L. Mills

ISBN: 978-1-63321-980-9

Chapter 5

Nystagmus in Posterior Fossa Stroke Patients

Ksenija Ribarić Jankes[1], Ljiljana Beslać Bumbaširević[2], Ivana Berisavac[3] and Višnja Padjen[4]
[1]Euromedik Hospital, Belgrade, Serbia
[2,3,4]Neurological Emergency Department, Stroke Unit, Emergency Centre of Serbia, Neurological Clinic, Clinical Center of Serbia, Belgrade, Medical Faculty Belgrade, Serbia

Introduction

In this chapter we will describe briefly the pathophysiological mechanisms of central nystagmus generation, proceed with the description of bedside examination of the patient with sudden onset of vertigo and unsteadiness. We will present the results of 9 patients with stroke diagnosis who were during the year 2013 admitted to our Neurological Emergency Department and who came with sudden onset of vertigo and unsteadiness as the leading symptom of illness. On the basis of these results we will discuss the importance of recognition of the impairment of central vestibular pathways as solely symptoms or additional symptoms in the early diagnosis of cerebral stroke. The therapeutic guidelines will be presented as well.

Pathophysiological Mechanisms of Central Nystagmus Generation

Vestibular pathways run from vestibular nerve and vestibular nuclei mostly through the fibers of medial longitudinal fasciculus (MLF) to the oculomotor nucleus and supranuclear integration centers in the midbrain (interstitial nucleus of Cajal (iC) and rostral interstitial medial longitudinal fasciculus (riMLF) nucleus).

Sometimes pathophysiology of the anatomical structures can explain the visible nystagmus but occasionally the topography of the nystagmus generation is not so simple. Nevertheless, we will try to present the pathophysiological mechanisms which lead to the generation of central vestibular nystagmus.

Gaze Holding

To start an eye movement, a burst of activity from motoneurons is needed. To maintain the gaze in one position, activity from neurons which differ cytoarchitecturally from motoneurons is necessary. Those neurons provide a constant tonic input to the ocular muscles and they are involved in gaze-holding. They form the so called neural integrator and additional clusters of cells which are interspread between and around the fasciculus of MLF [1] The neural integrator for horizontal eye movements is located in the vestibular nucleus/nucleus prepositus hypoglossi complex [2, 3]. Cell clusters around the crossing of the MLF fibers in lower pons (paramedial pontine reticular formation (PPRF)) are demonstrated to be involved in gaze holding as well [4]. In addition, the flocculus of the cerebellum supports gaze holding. For vertical gaze holding the (iC) in the mesencephalon is proved to be responsible [5].

If maintenance of stable conjugate eye deviation away from the primary position is not possible, the eyes drift back to the center and a corrective saccade (or fast phase) brings the eye back to the desired position. This happens for as long as the attempt of holding the eyes fixed on one object in the lateral position is present. The result is gaze-evoked nystagmus. The gaze evoked nystagmus changes it's direction with the change of gaze position. It is always present in the direction of gaze (Figure 1). The gaze evoked nystagmus generally appears on attempted gaze, but it can also occur spontaneously because of the difference between the null and the midposition of the eye.

Internuclear ophthalmoplegia (INO) is a pathologial oculomotor sign attributed to unilateral or bilateral MLF lesions. It is characterized by slowing of adduction of the eye on the side of the lesion and a gaze evoked nystagmus of the contralateral eye. INO can be present bilaterally [6]. The slowing of adduction is better visible in cases of larger compared to smaller lesions.

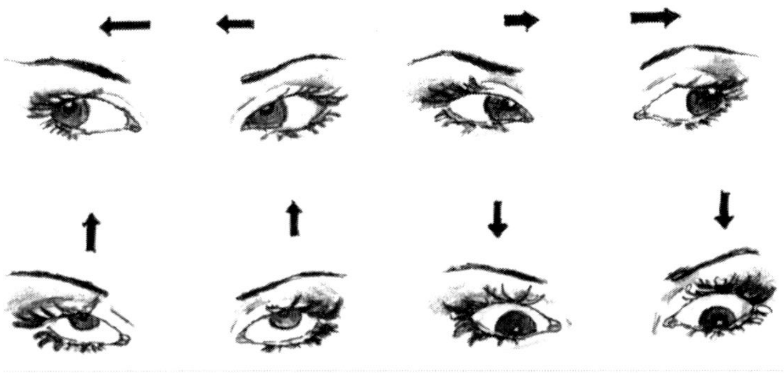

Figure 1. Gaze evoked nystagmus to the right, to the left, upwards and downwards. Arrows show the direction of eye movements and the amplitude of the movement of each eye.

Yaw, Roll and Pitch Plane

According to Brandt and Dieterich [7] signs and symptoms of vestibular dysfunction can be divided according to three planes of action of the vestibuloocular reflex (VOR): yaw, roll and pitch plane.

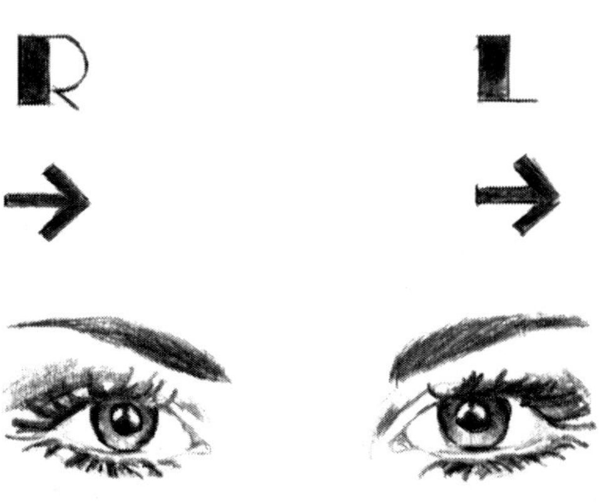

Figure 2. Horizontal nystagmus to the left, the arrows show that both eyes are moving with the same amplitude and in the same direction.

Spontaneous horizontal nystagmus is a VOR dysfunction in yaw plane (Figure 2). In most cases it is caused by the lesion of vestibular sense organ or nerve. It is rarely caused by central lesions but it can be present if the lesion involves a small part of the medial and superior vestibular nuclei and the adjacent centers for gaze holding (PPRF). Postural signs in the same plane are lateral head tilt and lateral body tilt toward the side of the lesion.

Roll Plane

If a unilateral central lesion of the vestibular afferent pathways happens, it mostly affects the so called graviceptive pathways which transduce the information from vertical semicircular canals and otoliths. The result is an imbalance of the vestibular input (tone imbalance) in the roll plane with a torsional nystagmus (Figure 3).

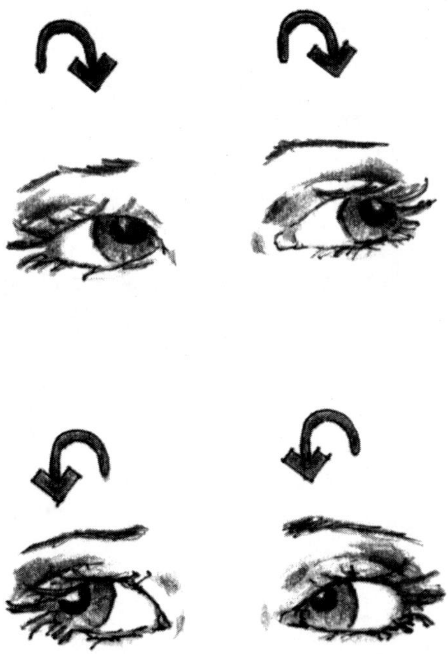

Figure 3. Torsional nystagmus. The arrows show the direction of eye movements.

Lesions of iC cause an ipsiversional torsional nystagmus while lesion of riMLF nucleus is responsible for a contralateral torsional nystagmus [8].

Postural signs are head and body tilt to the side opposite to the lesion, sometimes skew deviation with the undermost eye on the side opposite to the lesion and ocular torsion (Figure 4). Skew deviation can also accompany peripheral vestibular lesion of utricle [9]. Ocular torsion is present, but it can not be seen by bedside examination. It can be demonstrated by fundus photography. Therefore we will not discuss this symptom further. The triad of symptoms head tilt, skew deviation and ocular torsion is called ocular tilt reaction (OTR). It can be present some peripheral as well as central lesions of the vestibular pathways up to the mesencephalon.

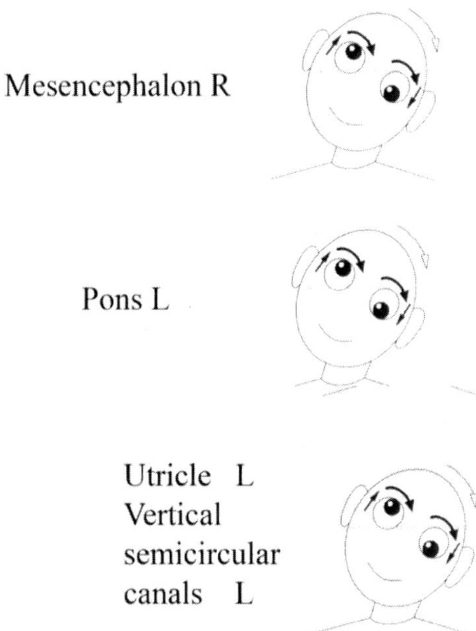

Figure 4. A shematic drowing of the vestibular syndromes in roll plane. On the labyrinthine and pontine level, head tilt and skew deviation are toward the lesion side, on the mezencephalic level they are toward the contralateral side (according to Brandt and Dieterich 1995).

Pitch Plane

Bilateral lesions of the central vestibular pathways result in vertical upbit nystagmus (pitch plane) and forward or backward body tilt.

Flocculus

Flocculus of the cerebellum supports the gaze holding, unilateral lesions of flocculus and its connections to the vestibular nuclei result in gaze holding deficit (Buettner and Grundei 1994) and failure of fixation suppression of the vestibular nystagmus [10]. Bilateral lesions of flocculus result in downbeat nystagmus.

Bedside Examination

Only neurootological tests which can enlarge the examination done by neurologist, and only the tests which can be done on bedside will be discussed. Various very useful neurootological tests for which some instruments are needed, will be skipped. The performance of tests already described in details previously in this book will not be repeated.

The spontaneous nystagmus caused by a damage or irritation of the vestibular apparatus/nerve was already previously described. If the eye movements are horizontal, our attendance must be directed to both eyes because if both eyes are moving with the same amplitude and in the same direction, we can call it horizontal "vestibular" nystagmus (figure No 2). If both eyes a moving spontaneously with torsion of both eyes in one direction, it is the spontaneous torsional nystagmus (figure No 3). If the eyes are moving spontaneously up or spontaneously down, this is the spontaneous vertical nystagmus. If the eyes are not moving spontaneously at the moment of examination, we provoke the nystagmus by positional tests. The horizontal vestibular nystagmus can be provoked also if the patient fixate on a target 30° to the right and then to the left. The nystagmus will occur only in one direction and both eyes will still be moving with the same amplitude (according to Alexander's I degree).

The next test used to provoke a horizontal "vestibular" nystagmus is the head shaking test. Nystagmus duration depends on the magnitude of the vestibular damage.

Next we try to provoke the gaze evoked nystagmus. The patient fixate on a target 30° to the left, to the right, up and down. The nystagmus which appears on gaze fixation is called the gaze evoked nystagmus. Usually with horizontal gaze fixation the amplitude of the abducted eye is larger then the amplitude of the adducted eye (figure No 2). The nystagmus changes it's direction with the direction of gaze. If the patient moves his abducted eye about 40° laterally the so called end point nystagmus can occur which is not a sign of illness. This nystagmus usually stops after a few second. Asking the patient to fixate his gaze at this position, we can sometimes discover a gaze evoked nystagmus which is a remnant of a previous illness of the peripheral or central vestibular pathways. The gaze evoked nystagmus can be caused by the damage of flocculo-vestibular connections. It changes the direction with the direction of gaze. According to our personal observations, in this case the evoked nystagmus is with equal amplitudes on both eyes, usually with low frequency. For this observation we don't have any experimental confirmation. Vertical fixational nystagmus appears at upward or downward gaze fixation. More often is the upward nystagmus.

Skew Deviation

By horizontal head impuls (or head thrust) test a recent horizontal canal paresis can be demonstrated. The observer can be uncertain about the result in the case of mild or moderate lateral canal paresis.

Caloric test is the other way to test if canal paresis exists. The standard bitermal caloric test with hot (44°) and cold (30°) water can not be easily performed at bedside. Therefore we use the test described by Torok. The test is done first with a weak stimulus (10 ml) and then with a strong stimulus (100 ml) of 20° cold water. The postcaloric nystagmus duration is measured in seconds. The postcaloric nystagmus lasts for about 50 seconds after weak stimulus application, and about 90 seconds after the strong stimulus application. If a more then 25% asymmetry between the left and the right side exists, the patient suffers of a horizontal canal paresis [11]. The general recomendation for the time of caloric test accomplishment is more then 4 days after beginning of sudden vertigo.

The Vestibulospinal Tests

The past pointing test is positive in terms of deviation of the arm to one side during the attempt to touch the examiners finger with closed eyes. It is a nice demonstration of hypotonia of arm muscles after sudden impairment of the vestibular apparatus. Romberg test and "sharpened" Romberg test although not specific for vestibular instability, can be used at the beginning of the illness when a clear inclination or swaying to one side can be demonstrated. During the "sharpened" Romberg test the patient stand in the tandem heel-to-toe position with eyes closed and arms folded against the chest. He inclines or falls toward the impaired side.

Tandem walking (heal-to-toe) is not possible in acute vestibular illness.

Methods

We performed a retrospective study of 723 in-patients of our Neurological Emergency Department admitted to the Department during the year 2013. There were 53% of women, 47% of men, between 18 and 78 years (mean 42 years). The patients with sudden vertigo and sudden instability as the dominant symptom of illness were selected. Patients with vertigo and hearing loss were excluded from this study. All patients where first seen by a neurologist. A computerized tomography (CT) scan was performed before the admission and repeated within 22 to 36 hours, or earlier, in cases of clinical deterioration. In some patients a diffusion weighted magnetic resonance imaging was performed (MR) as additional neuroimaging tool. Each patient with vertigo was also seen by a ENT specialist-neurotologist, on the first or on the second day of admission.

In all patients with suspected stroke, the evaluation of blood vessels of head and neck was done by using Carotid Doppler Sonography (CDS), Transcranial Doppler (TCD) and CT angiography.

Therapeutic process for patients with suspected stroke included their treatment in the stroke unit following the protocol which was made based on recommendation of current guidelines [12, 13].

Results

Out of 723 in-patients, only 22 were hospitalized because of sudden vertigo and sudden instability as the dominant symptom of illness. After precise clinical examination, 9 patients were diagnosed as cerebral stroke, 13 as vestibular neuronitis.

The results of the patients with stroke are shown on Table 1. The patients were between 26 and 75 years old, 5 female, 4 male. CT scan was done in all of them at the moment of admission, and was repeated in following 22-36 hours from the symptom onset. MR was done in 5 patients.

Table 1.

Name	Years	Imaging	Diagnosis	Additional neurological signs	Neurotological signs
M.S.	54	MR and CT	Cerbll inf R Sten vert a R	Yes	spont H ny to the L HIT: paresis R cal test: paresis R FFS R side vest spin tests: inclination to the R
M.M.	75	CT	Pontin inf L and cerbll inf R	Yes	paresis n. VI L gaze evok ny to R HIT: uncertain cal test: symmet vest spin tests: without incl to one side
K.S.	54	CT	Cerbll inf R Ocl vert a R	Yes	gaze evok ny to the R HIT: symmet cal test: symmet FFS on the R vest spin tests: ataxia
V.M.	73	CT	Cerbll inf L	No	gaze evok ny to the R and to the L HIT: symmet cal test: symetr with FFS bil vest spin tests: ataxia
V.D.	45	MR	Mezenceph inf L	Yes	Spont torsional ny to the R Skew dev with the lower R eye HIT: uncertain cal test: symmet vest. spin tests: incl. to R
D.B.	53	MR	Thalam inf L Sy trunci cerebri	Yes	Paresis n. VI L gaze evok ny to the R HIT: symmet cal test:symmet vest. spin tests: incl L
M.M.	61	MR	Pontine inf R Ocl vert a R	Yes	INO R HIT: uncertain cal test: not performed vest spin tests: not performed
N.J.	26	MR	Mezencephalic inf L	No	Spont torsional to the R Haed tilt R HIT: uncertain cal test: symmet vest. spin tests: incl to the R
K.S.	55	CT	Cerbll inf R Sten vert a R	Yes	Gaze evok ny to R HIT: symmet vest. spin tests: ataxia

Cerbll - cerebellar, inf - infarction, R - right, sten - stenosis, vert -vertebral, a - artery, L - left, ocl - occlusion, mezenceph - mezencephalic, Thalam - Thalamic, Sy - syndroma, Midbr - Midbrain, spont - spontaneous, H - horizontal, ny - nystagmus, HIT - head impuls test, cal - caloric, FFS - failure of fixation suppression, vest spin – vestibulospinal, gaze evok – gaze evoked, symmet – symmetrical, incl – inclination, dev – deviation.

Isolated cerebellar infarction was present in 4 patients, pontine and cerebellar infarction in 1 patient. Isolated pontine infarction in 1, mezencephalic infarction in two patients, thalamic infarction together with brainstem syndrome in one.

Unilateral stenosis or oclusion of vertebral artery was demonstrated in fore patients (3 with cerebellar infarction, 1 with pontine infarction). Neurotological finding is listed in details. Exept neurotological positive finding, additional neurological signs (involvement of long pathways, other cranial nerve (exept vest. nerve and abducens nerve) lesions, hemihipesthesia, dismetria) were present in 7 patients, in two they were not.

Spontaneous horizontal nystagmus was present in one patient, peripheral vestibular ethiology was demonstrated by head impuls test (HIT) and caloric testing, as well as by vestibulospinal tests (toward one side). The cerebellar involvement was demonstrated with unilateral failure of fixation suppression (FFS).

Spontaneous torsional nystagmus was present in two patients. One had torsional ny to the left side, skew deviation with the lower right eye, inclination to the right while performing the vestibulospinal tests, symmetrical HIT and symmetrical caloric test. The other had spontaneous torsional nystagmus to the right, head tilt to the left and inclination to the left while performing the vestibulospinal tests. HIT was symetrical as well as the caloric test.

Three patients with cerebellar infarction had gaze evoked nystagmus: one bilateral while two to the side of cerebellar lesion. HIT and the caloric test were symetrical in all three patients. One had bilateral FFS, the other two unilateral, on the side of cerebellar lesion. Ataxia was present in all patients while performing the vestibulospinal tests.

The patient with pontine and cerebellar lesion had abducens nerve paresis on the left side and gaze evoked nystagmus to the right. HIT was uncertain, caloric test symetrical, and he did not incline to one side while performing the vestibulospinal tests.

One patient had isolated pontine lesion on the right side. Internuclear ophtalmoplegia (INO) was present at the side of lesion. HIT was judged as uncertain. Caloric test and vestibulospinal tests were not performed because patient's general condition worsened.

In one patient a thalamic infarction was visible with MR, but clinical examination demonstrated that a brainstem syndrome is present in addition. An abducens nerve paresis was present on the left side, a gaze evoked nystagmus on the right side. HIT was symetrical, caloric test symetrical, during the vestibulospinal tests he inclined to the left.

Therapy

Only 1 of 9 patients arrived at the hospital within the therapeutic window of 4.5 hours for administration of intravenous thrombolytic therapy and was consequently treated with it. The secondary stroke prevention was done by using Aspirin, dose 300 mg, which was introduced in the first 48 hours from symptoms onset. Patients were also treated with intravenous solution (0.9% Sodium Chloride and Ringer) as well as antiemetic, and other therapy for control of cerebrovascular risk factors.

Discussion

To recognize the impairment of central vestibular pathways in patient with sudden onset of vertigo and unsteadiness is of crucial importance in neurological practice, especially in Neurological Emergency Units.

During last few years the importance of this recognition was stressed in several publications (14, 15, 16, 17).

Among 723 patients hospitalized at Emergency Neurology Department of Clinical Centre of Serbia, 22 came with sudden vertigo and unsteadiness as a leading symptom of their illness.

Thirteen of them were diagnosed as vestibular neuritis and treated accordingly. Nine of them were diagnosed as cerebral stroke. We analyzed which neurotological signs accompanied which localization of stroke and how effective single diagnostic procedures were in establishing the diagnosis.

In cerebellar stroke patients, only one patient had a peripheral vestibular impairment additionally. This impairment was recognized by typical signs of peripheral vestibular damage: horizontal nystagmus, positive HIT, body inclination toward the lesion side, unilateral paresis in caloric test. The cerebellar sign was in this case the unilateral FFS. Besides neurotological, the patient had neurological signs as explained on the table. The neurotological signs demonstrated at the bedside, that a peripheral vestibular damage is present, signs of cerebellar involvement were revealed after a few days when the caloric test was performed. In this case, crucial for the stroke diagnosis was the neurological examination.

Three other patients with cerebellar stroke had the unilateral or bilateral gaze-evoked nystagmus. Two of them had unilateral or bilateral FFS. In two patients with cerebellar stroke additional neurological signs were present. In one patient neurological signs were not present, the only neurotological sign of central impairment was gaze evoked nystagmus. On the basis of this sign, the CT imaging was performed and stroke was revealed. Therefore, we underline that gaze evoked nystagmus is an important sign of the damage of central vestibular pathways (in this case probably cerebello-vestibular connections).

The first patient with mezencephalic infarction, had typical symptoms: spontaneous torsional ny to the left, skew deviation with the lower R eye, simetrical caloric test, body inclination to the R. Additional neurological sign were present.

The second patient with mezencephalic infarction, a young woman of 28 years, only a spontaneous torsional nystagmus to the right was present together with the head tilt to the right. None of additional neurological signs were present. In this patient, the suspicion of brain stroke was raised only on the basis of neurotological signs, and with MR imaging, the suspicion was confirmed.

In patients with pontine infarction the central vestibular signs were typical: INO and abducens paresis with gaze evoked nystagmus to the opposite side.

The greatest importance of central vestibular pathways impairment recognition is in patients who don't have additional neurological signs. This was the case in our two patients (one with cerebellar and one with mezencephalic stroke). Grace to this recognition, the proper therapy was immediately administered and all possible risk factor were explored in order of second stroke prevention.

Kattah and coworkers (17) introduced the acronym of HINTS for head impuls, nystagmus and test of skew, as the most important steps of bedside oculomotor examination (in differentiation between the periferal vestibular impairment and stroke). The group of Kattah and coworkers observed the skew deviation by means of prism cross cover test. In our patients skew deviation judgement was not done by prism cross cover test, therefore we can not comment their finding of skew deviation. However with a small number of patients with brainstem lesion, we would not expect a greater percentage of skew. We confirm the importance of the given acronym. In our patients, besides the gaze evoked nystagmus, an important diagnostic sign was FFS which discovered cerebellar dysfunction.

Acknowledgments

We are grateful for the extensive technical help to MSc Ljubomir Damjanović, for figure drawings to Misses Maja Pecić Ristić and for the additional technical help to MSc Vuk Ađić.

References

[1] Buettner-Ennever JA, Horn AKE, Schmidtke K. Cell groups of medial longitudinal f and paramedian tractsasciculus. *Rev. Neurol.* (Paris) 1989;145,8-9:533-539.

[2] Robinson DA. Integrating with neurons. *Annu. Rev. Neurosci.* 1989; 12:33-45.

[3] Buettner U, Grundei T. Gaze-evoked nystagmus and smooth pursuit deficits: their relationship studied in 52 patients. *J. Neurol.* 1995;242:384-389.

[4] Bronstein AM, Rudge P, Gresty MA, Boulay G Du, Morris Joan. Abnormalities of horizontal gaze. Clinical, oculographic and magnetic tesonance imaging findings. II Gaze palsy and internuclear ophthalmoplegia. *Journal of Neurology, Neurosurgery and Psychiatry* 1990; 53:200-207.

[5] Crawford JD, Cadera W, Vilis T. Generation of torsional and vertical eye position signals by the interstitial nucleus of Cajal. *Science* 1991;252:1551-1553.

[6] Bird AC, Leech J. Internuclear ophthalmoplegia. *Brit. J. Ophthal.* 1976;60:645-651.

[7] Brandt Th, Dieterich M. Central vestibular syndromes in roll, pitch and yaw planes. *Neuro-ophthalmology* 1995;15(6):291-303.

[8] Helmchen C, Rambold H, Kempermann U, Buettner-Ennever JA, Buettner U. Localizing value of torsional nystagmus in small midbrain lesions. *Neurology* 2002;59:1956-1964.

[9] Halmaghy GM, Gresty MA, Gibson WPR. Ocular tilt reaction with peripheral vestibular lesion. *Ann. Neurol.* 1979;6:80-83.

[10] Kato I, Sato Y, Aoyagi M, Mizukoshi K, Kimura Y, Koike Y, Hayano N. Caloric paern test with special reference to failure of fixation-supression. *Acta Otolaryngol.* 1979;88:97-104.

[11] Ribarić-Jankes K, Čobeljić R, Svetel M, Pešić B. Vestibular function after spinal cord injury: preliminary results. *Spinal Cord* 2009;47:401-404.

[12] The European Stroke Organization (ESO) Executive Committe and the ESO Writing Committee. Guidelines for management of ischemic stroke and transient ischemic attack 2008. *Cerebrovasc. Dis.* 2008;25:457-507.

[13] Guidelines for the Early management of Patients With Acute Ischemic Stroke. A Guideline for Healthcare Professionals From the American Heart Association/American Stroke Association. *Stroke* 2013;44:870-947.

[14] Newman-Toker DE, Hsieh YH, Camargo CA Jr, Pelletier AJ,Butshy GT, Edlow JA. Spectrumm of dizzeness visits to US emergency departments: cross sectional analysis from a nationally representative simple. *Mayo Clin. Proc.* 2008;83:765-775.

[15] Chase M, Joyce NR, Carney E, Salciccioli JD, Vinton D, Donnino MW, Edlow JA. ED patients with vertigo: dan we identify clinical factors associated with acute stroke? *Am. J. Emerg. Med.* 2012;30(4):587-591.

[16] Newman-Toker DE, Camargo CA Jr, Hsieh YH,Pelleier AJ, Edlow JA. Disconnect between charted vestibular diagnoses and emergency department management decisions: a cross-sectional analysis from a nationally representative sample. *Acad. Emerg. Med.* 2009;16(10):970-977.

[17] Kattah JC, Talkad AV, Wang DZ, Hsieh Yu-H, Newman-Toker DE. HINTS to Diagnose Stroke in the Acute Vestibular Syndrome: Three-Step Bedside Oculomotor Examination More Sensitive Than Early MRI Diffusion-Weighted Imaging. *Stroke* 2009;40:3504-3510.

Index

A

B

C

D

E

F

G

H

O

P

Q

R

S

T

U

V

W